AF251905

Multi-Level Mammaplasty

*Anatomical Support and
Re-Shaping of the Breast*

Multi-Level Mammaplasty

Anatomical Support and Re-Shaping of the Breast

Amiram Borenstein

Borenstein Plastic Surgery Clinic, Israel

Or Friedman

Suckler Faculty of Medicine, Israel

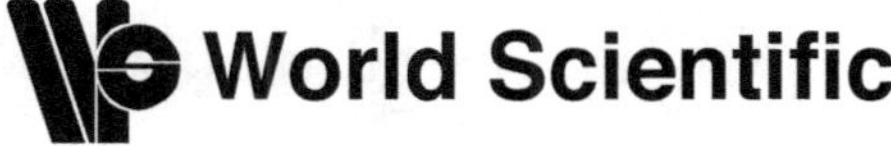

World Scientific

NEW JERSEY · LONDON · SINGAPORE · BEIJING · SHANGHAI · HONG KONG · TAIPEI · CHENNAI · TOKYO

Published by

World Scientific Publishing Co. Pte. Ltd.

5 Toh Tuck Link, Singapore 596224

USA office: 27 Warren Street, Suite 401-402, Hackensack, NJ 07601

UK office: 57 Shelton Street, Covent Garden, London WC2H 9HE

British Library Cataloguing-in-Publication Data
A catalogue record for this book is available from the British Library.

MULTI-LEVEL MAMMAPLASTY
Anatomical Support and Re-Shaping of the Breast

ISBN 978-981-121-912-2 (hardcover)
ISBN 978-981-121-913-9 (ebook for institutions)
ISBN 978-981-121-914-6 (ebook for individuals)

For any available supplementary material, please visit
https://www.worldscientific.com/worldscibooks/10.1142/11792#t=suppl

DEDICATION

To Muriel Borenstein my lovely wife who has accompanied me from the very start of this journey.

To Offer Friedman and Benny Mandel for their guidance and endless support.

CONTENTS

List of Figures — xi

Preface — Short Scar Mammaplasty Evolution — xiii

Acknowledgments — xvii

Chapter 1 **Surgical Anatomy of the Breast** — 1

The Superficial Fascia of the Breast — 1
Blood Supply — 3
Innervation — 7

Chapter 2 **Multi-Level Mammaplasty** — 9

Fundamentals — 9
Surgical Principles of Multi-level Mammaplasty — 10
Upper pole — 10
Inferior pole — 10
Multi-level breast mound support — 12
Nipple–areola placement — 12
Tension-free skin closure — 12
Symmetry, scars, safety, and stability of results — 12
Scars — 14
Sensitivity — 14
Lactation potential — 14
Adaptability — 14

Chapter 3 **Patient Consultation and Evaluation** — 17

Go On, I Am Listening — 17
Consultation, Motivations, and Indications — 17
Medical History and Physical Examination — 19
Informing the Patient — 20

Chapter 4 **Multi-Level Breast Reduction** — 23

Secure the Foundation — 23
Surgical Technique and Rationale — 23

Marking and de-epithelization 23
Lateral support 24
Shaping the breast mound 28
Nipple–areola complex insetting 28
What About Mastopexy? 34
Concluding Thoughts 35
Tips and Tricks to the Technique 38
Limitations 39
Summary 39

Chapter 5 Breast Implant Explantation and Multi-Level Mastopexy 41
Out With the Old (Implant) in With Your Own (Breast) 41
Surgical Technique 41
Discussion 44
Tips and Tricks to the Technique 44
Limitations 47
Conclusion 47

Chapter 6 Breast Augmentation and Multi-Level Mastopexy 49
Taking the Stress Out of the Breast 49
Surgical Technique 49
Discussion 55
Tips and Tricks to the Technique 56
Limitations 57
Conclusion 57

Chapter 7 Postoperational Breast Support 59
The Paper Bra 59
Breast Taping Technique 59
Follow-up 61
Discussion 62
Limitations 62
Conclusion 62

Chapter 8 Complications and Long-Term Results 63
Stand By Me 63
General Considerations 63
Necrosis 63
Infection hematoma and seroma 64
Wound dehiscence 65
Delayed Problem 65
Poor healing and scarring 65
Long-term results 65

Chapter 9   Advanced Scar Treatments   67

    Scars Are Like Diamonds   67
        Scar Treatment   67
        Mature and Stable Surgical Scars   68
        Erythematous and Relatively Flat Surgical Scars   68
        Erythematous and Slightly Hypertrophic Post-surgical Scars   69
        Mature/Stable (Non-Erythematous) Hypertrophic Scars   69
        Atrophic Scars   69
        Hyperpigmented Scars   70
        Hypopigmented Scars   72
        Immature Scar or Scar Mitigation   72
        Conclusion   73

References   75

List of Abbreviations   81

Index   83

LIST OF FIGURES

Figure 1.   Scar extending to chest wall   xiv
Figure 2.   Illustration of the multi-level mammaplasty technique   xv
Figure 1.1.   Deep musculature of the breast   2
Figure 1.2.   Superficial fascia system   3
Figure 1.3.   Arterial blood supply to the breast   4
Figure 1.4.   Arterial blood supply to the deep central breast tissue   5
Figure 1.5.   Arterial blood supply to the breast   6
Figure 1.6.   Breast innervation   7
Figure 1.7.   Breast innervation   8
Figure 2.1.   Multi-level mammaplasty   10
Figure 2.2.   Upper pole   11
Figure 2.3.   Lower pole   11
Figure 2.4.   The multi-level mammaplasty from bird's eye view   13
Figure 2.5.   Tension-free skin closure   14
Figure 3.1.   Natural progression of breast descent after surgery   21
Figure 4.1.   Marking the future nipple–areola complex position   24
Figure 4.2.   Marking the expected de-epithelization and excision borders   25
Figure 4.3.   De-epithelization   26
Figure 4.4.   Lower pole tissue resection   26
Figure 4.5.   Undermining of the breast tissue   27
Figure 4.6.   Lateral sutures   27
Figure 4.7.   Pillar sutures   28
Figure 4.8.   Raising the skin flaps   29
Figure 4.9.   A single figure of 8 sutures   29
Figure 4.10.   Repeating the Borenstein maneuver   30
Figure 4.11.   Precise trimming of the skin   31
Figure 4.12.   Nipple-areola complex final de-epithelization   31
Figure 4.13.   Nipple-areola complex (NAC) placement   32
Figure 4.14.   Paper bra postsurgical dressing technique   33
Figure 4.15.   Treatment of large ptotic breast   34
Figure 4.16.   Overly large breast reduction   36
Figure 4.17.   Treatment of large and asymmetric breasts   37

Figure 5.1.   Explantation pexy markings, de-epithelization, and incision   42
Figure 5.2.   Explantation pexy removal of implant   43
Figure 5.3.   Explantation pexy restructuring the breast   45
Figure 5.4.   Borenstein explantation–pexy technique   46
Figure 5.5.   Borenstein explantation–pexy technique   47
Figure 5.6.   Borenstein explantation–pexy technique   48
Figure 5.7.   Borenstein explantation–pexy technique   48
Figure 6.1.   Borenstein augmentation–pexy technique   50
Figure 6.2.   Borenstein augmentation–pexy technique   51
Figure 6.3.   Borenstein augmentation–pexy technique   52
Figure 6.4.   Borenstein augmentation–pexy technique   53
Figure 6.5.   Borenstein augmentation–pexy technique   54
Figure 6.6.   Borenstein augmentation–pexy technique   55
Figure 6.7.   Borenstein augmentation–pexy technique   56
Figure 6.8.   Borenstein augmentation–pexy technique   57
Figure 7.1.   Paper bra technique   60
Figure 7.2.   Paper bra removal   61
Figure 8.1.   Borenstein breast reduction   65
Figure 8.2.   Borenstein breast reduction   66
Figure 8.3.   Borenstein breast reduction   66
Figure 9.1.   Treatment of a mature stable scar   68
Figure 9.2.   Treatment of erythematous and relatively flat surgical scars   69
Figure 9.3.   Treatment of erythematous and hypertrophic surgical scars   70
Figure 9.4.   Treatment of atrophic surgical scars   71
Figure 9.5.   Treatment of hyperpigmented surgical scars   71
Figure 9.6.   Treatment of an immature surgical scar   72

PREFACE — SHORT SCAR MAMMAPLASTY EVOLUTION

Patients seeking breast reduction or mastopexy vary substantially. Common medical complaints include limitation of sports activity, back pain, inframammary fold (IMF) fungal infection, intertrigo, irritation, and even abrasion wounds from the bra suspenders on the shoulders.[1] Most of our patients claim they do not like their breasts. Some patients avoid swimwear, have difficulties shopping for bras, or merely wish they could wear a buttoned blouse.

Several landmark evolutions in breast reduction technique influenced how most surgeons approach mammaplasty today. The vertical scar technique for reduction mammaplasty was first described in 1925, but popularized by Claude Lassus in 1964, and soon after, modified by Madeleine Lejour, limiting the scar to a vertical pattern.[2] The vertical skin incision pattern has been adapted to inferior, medial, superomedial, and lateral pedicles.[3] In parallel, in 1956, Robert Wise described a skin resection pattern, adapted from a brassiere design, which became known as the inverted T. Ivo Pitanguy introduced the superior pedicle technique during the 1960s.[3–8]

Most traditional reduction mammaplasty or mastopexy techniques result in a visible submammary scar, if the incisions extend along the sides of the breast.[9] Surgeons have attempted to reduce the length of the incision, implementing short submammary scar techniques, though with varying degrees of success. Some surgeons eliminated the medial leg of the incision, creating a J or an L scar.[10–13] Others have used the inverted T incision but shortened the horizontal leg.[14,15] However, most of these techniques are applicable only in patients with small- to moderate-sized breasts.

Dartigues (1925) was the first to propose a vertical subareolar skin and glandular excision through a single vertical incision, without a horizontal submammary extension.[16] This technique was mainly intended for patients with moderate breast ptosis and hypertrophy.[16] Arie (1957) expanded the application of the Dartigues operation to include patients with larger breasts. In these patients, he raised the skin of the entire breast before reshaping the breast, fixed the reshaped breast to the periosteum of the ribs, and closed with a vertical suture that crossed the submammary fold.[17]

Although Arie's technique was popular in South America and became known worldwide through Converse's book *Reconstructive Plastic Surgery: Principles and Procedures in Correction, Reconstruction and Transplantation,*[18] its application was mainly appropriate for the correction of minor hypertrophy, since the vertical scar crossed the submammary fold and was visible when a two-piece bathing suit was worn.[18]

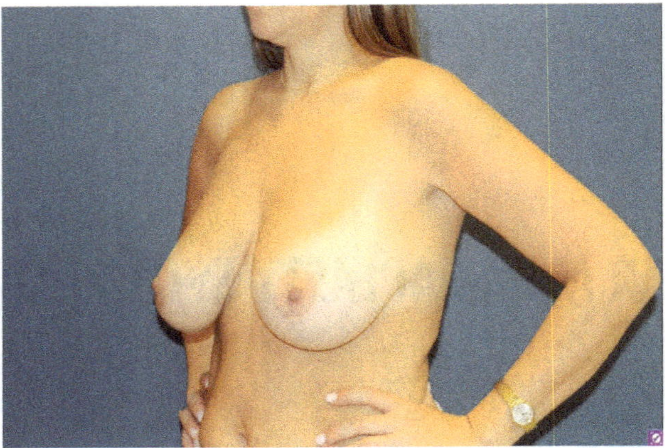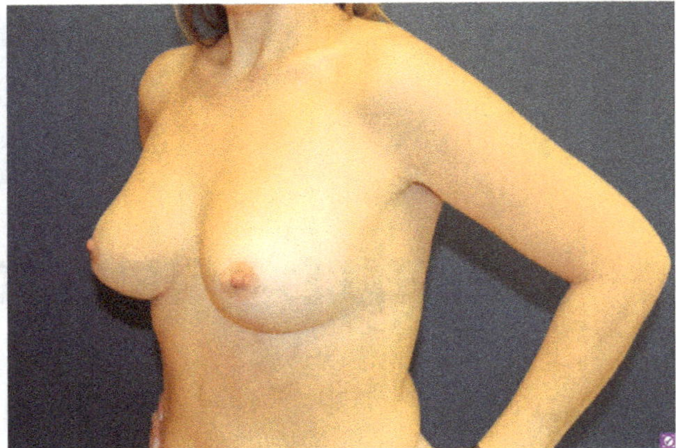

Figure 1. ■ Scar extending to chest wall. One year after surgery. On the left image, note the patient before surgery. On the right image, note the patient one year after surgery and the vertical scar extending beyond the IMF yet barely visible.

For example, an image of the scar extending to the chest wall, taken immediately after the surgery and one month later is shown in Fig. 1.

Usually, within the first month after surgery, breast appearance considerably improves due to scar retraction and descending of the breasts.

Lassus reintroduced the vertical mammaplasty technique in 1970, but abandoned it because of the unattractive lower extension of the vertical scar, opting instead for a short submammary scar technique.[14] In 1986, Lassus resumed the practice of the vertical mammaplasty technique, demonstrating that when the lower marking is placed above the submammary fold, the horizontal submammary scar can be avoided without creating a long vertical scar.[19]

The Borenstein Multi-level Mammaplasty: The focus of this book is, in fact, a modification of the Lassus technique, adjusted for use in breasts of all shapes and sizes. This method relies on an upper pedicle relative to the areola and involves a lower central breast reduction, glandular shaping, and suturing. The trade-off is that in order to ensure a fine-line peri-areolar scar, a vertical extension is added. However, this vertical scar fades over time and is partly obscured by the breast. The submammary horizontal scar, typical of the inverted T incision, is avoided by progressively gathering the breast tissue during the reconstruction of the breast mound, precisely trimming the excess skin for a short, tension-free vertical suture. Moreover, the peri-areolar suture is not disturbed by the vertical suture with unnecessary tension. Still, in the larger breast, the vertical scar may extend to the chest wall. We accept this trade-off and discuss it with our patients before surgery. In this book, we will present evidence to demonstrate that the Borenstein multi-level mammaplasty technique (Fig. 2) is safe and allows the precise reshaping of the breast with long-lasting results. Its advantages largely compensate for the addition of the vertical limb to the peri-areolar scar.

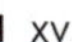

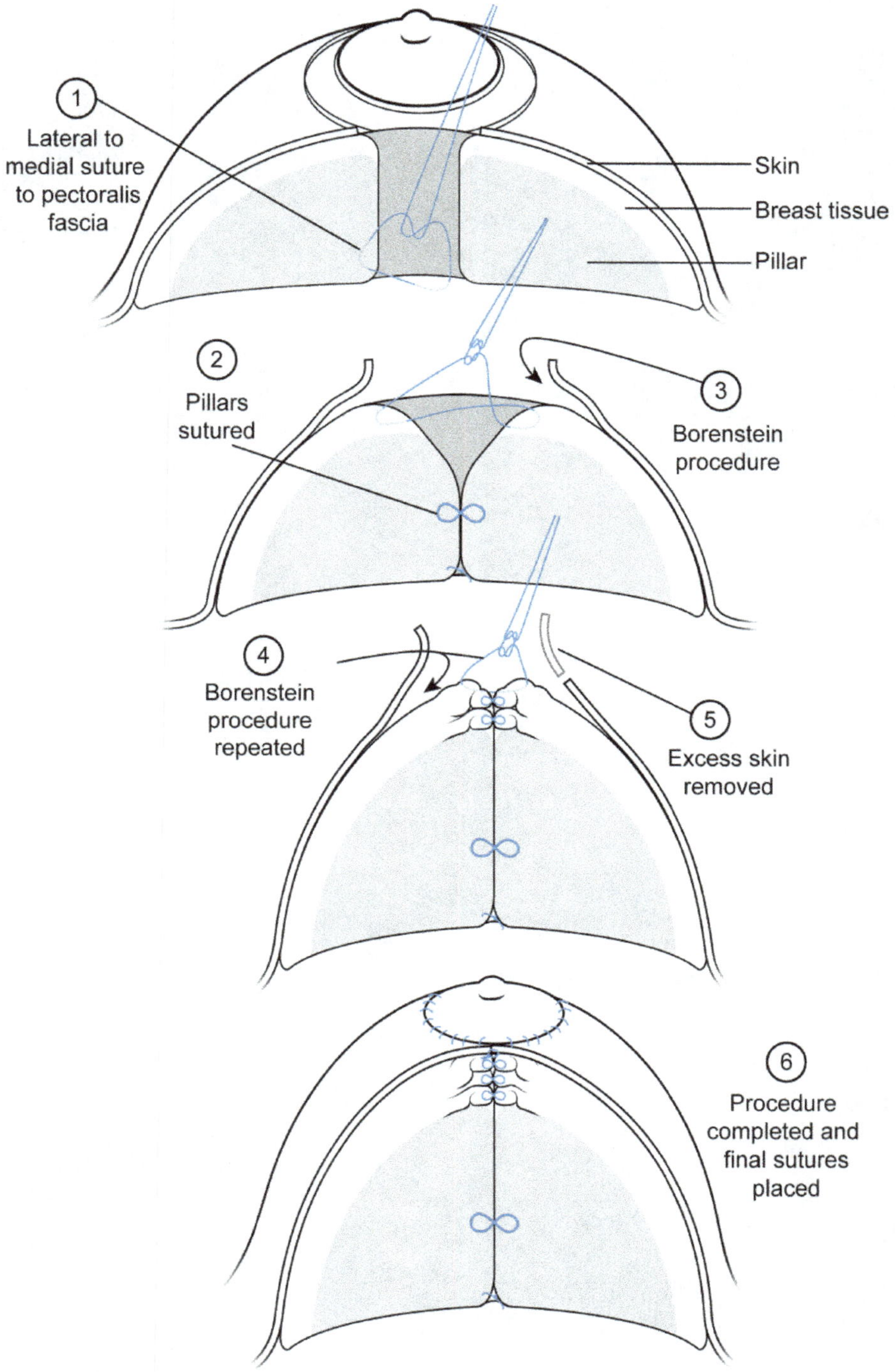

Figure 2. ■ Illustration of the multi-level mammaplasty technique.

ACKNOWLEDGMENTS

The preparation of this book was possible thanks to the tireless effort and support of our team: Romi Dahari and Sivan Bronstein, Yael Cohen, Nataly Afruz, Osnat Hauzi, and honorary member Igal Goldenberg.

They truly are the embodiment of Rudyard Kiplings words:

"If you can dream—and not make dreams your master;
If you can think—and not make thoughts your aim;
If you can meet with Triumph and Disaster
And treat those two impostors just the same;
If you can bear to hear the truth you've spoken
Twisted by knaves to make a trap for fools,
Or watch the things you gave your life to, broken,
And stoop and build 'em up with worn-out tools":

By Joseph Rudyard Kipling
("Brother Square-Toes"—Rewards and Fairies)

1

Surgical Anatomy of the Breast

The breast is typically described as extending from the second rib superiorly to the sixth rib inferiorly with the sternum located medially and the midaxillary line — laterally.

The human breast is a modified cutaneous exocrine gland, comprises the skin and the subcutaneous tissue. The breast gland comprises the ducts, lobules, and supporting stroma. Fat is interposed in a complex network of ligaments, nerves, arteries, veins, and lymphatics.[20]

The underlying breast tissue connects to the skin via an anterior fascial layer and the superficial fibrous extensions of Cooper ligaments, named after Sir Astley Cooper, who advanced the understanding of breast anatomy in his book *On the Anatomy of the Breast*, written in 1840.[21] The deep parenchymal tissues of the breast are enveloped by both the anterior and posterior fascial layers.[22] The breast overlies the pectoralis major muscle superiorly, the serratus anterior muscle laterally, and the upper abdominal oblique muscle inferiorly[22] (Fig. 1.1).

The only constant relationship of the breast with the underlying muscle is the submammary fold, which lies between the fifth and the eighth ribs and crosses one or two ribs obliquely.[23]

The true medial, lateral, and upper limits of the breast are the mobile landmarks, subject to modification without a need for reattachment or reconstruction.

These borders are easily identified by gently pressing the breast against the chest wall (Fig. 1.1) and noting the concave transition areas from breast mound convexity.

The Superficial Fascia of the Breast

A system of fascia surrounds the breast gland and encases it in two layers of fat and fascia. This is the superficial fascia system of the breast. The superficial layer is flimsy and easily overlooked during dissection. The deep layer is consistent in density and contributes to a gliding plane on the deep fascia that covers the underlying muscles.[24]

The anchorage of the superficial fascia system to the deep fascia of the chest at the breast's perimeter is the circummammary ligament. Specialized vertical cutaneous ligaments, known as the Cooper ligaments, travel from the posterior lamina fascia, through the breast gland and the anterior lamina, to anchor in the skin.[24] The circummammary ligament acts as the passage that arteries and nerves travel through, on their way to the breast parenchyma and the nipple–areola complex (NAC). The superficial fascia system is responsible for the shape of the breast.[23] The

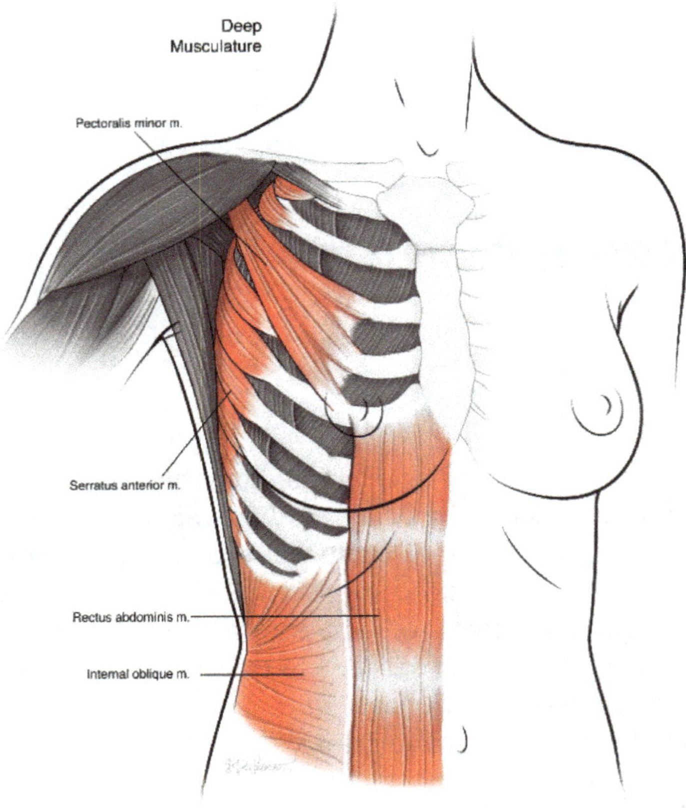

Figure 1.1. ■ **Deep musculature of the breast.** Note the anatomical relationship between the musculature and the bone foundation on which the breast mound is set.

fibrous attachments of the circummammary ligament are much stronger in the lower part of the breast than in the upper region, forming the submammary fold.[24] This landmark remains relatively stable throughout the patient's life.[24]

The strength of these deep attachments is apparent during mammaplasty when the central part of the gland is detached from the chest muscles starting inferiorly and moving upward. Under the lower part of the breast, this detachment cannot be performed with blunt finger dissection without injuring the underlying muscles. Higher on the pectoralis major muscle, however, separation is readily accomplished with blunt finger dissection in the loose areolar tissue that is located between these two fascial layers.

Stretching and relaxing of the superficial fascia system (Fig. 1.2), through aging or after surgery, along with variable amounts of support from the underlying chest wall, leads to breast ptosis. Intimate knowledge of this system is fundamental to both reconstructive and cosmetic breast surgeries.[25]

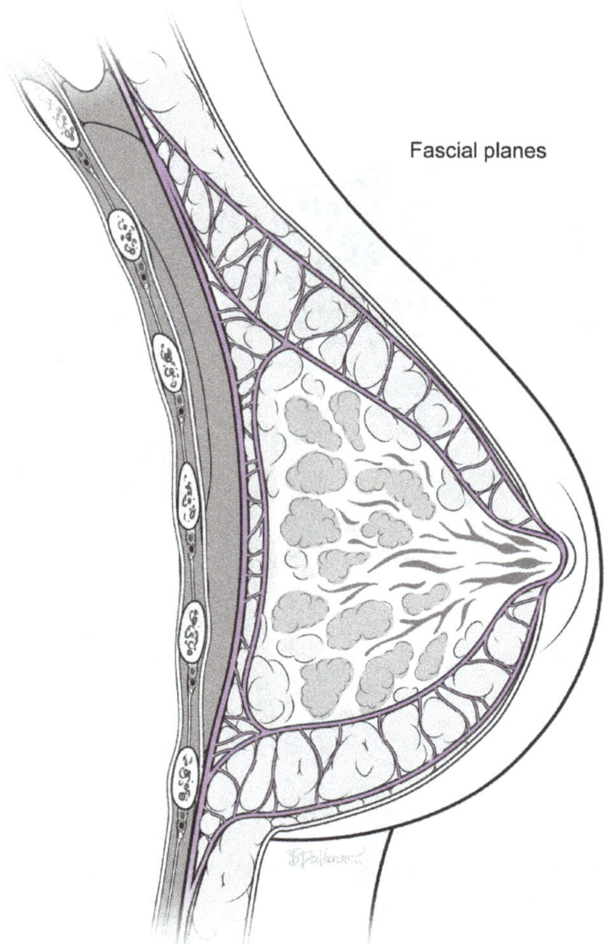

Figure 1.2. ■ **Superficial fascia system.** Note the bilayer structure surrounding the breast tissue. It is this structure that shapes the breast and it is this structure that we should use to support the new structure formed.

Blood Supply

The blood supply to the breast varies with age, hormonal status, and parenchymal breast volume. Premenopausal women typically have more blood volume in the breast as compared with postmenopausal women, with the largest concentration of blood vessels in the nipple.[26]

The arterial supply to the breast is primarily derived from branches of the internal thoracic (mammary) artery, the intercostal arteries, and the lateral thoracic artery (Fig. 1.3).

Superficially, the arterial branches of the internal and lateral thoracic arteries arborize across the breast and send perforating branches deep into the breast parenchyma. Along the posterior (deep) margin of the breast, branches of the intercostal arteries travel along with the pectoralis

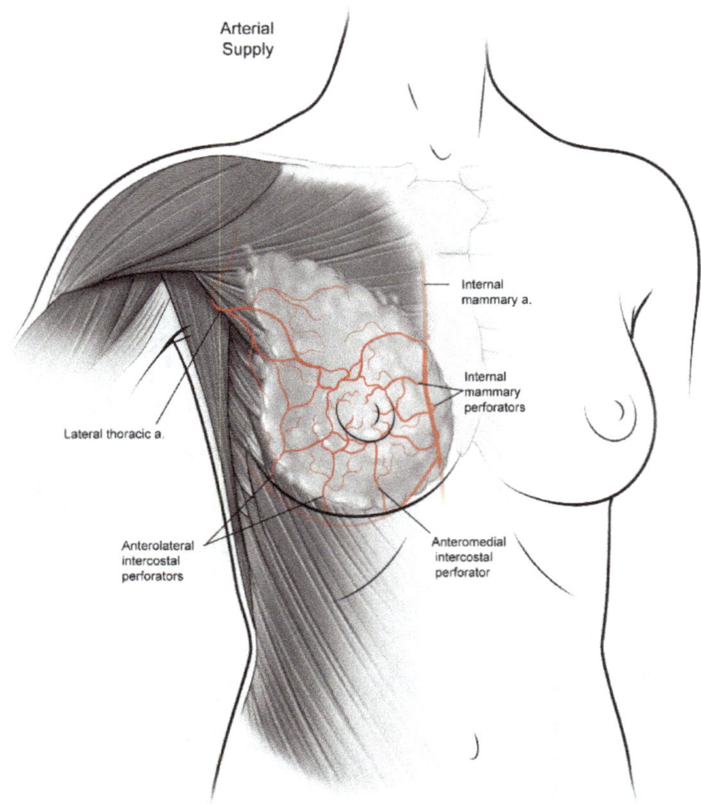

Figure 1.3. ■ Arterial blood supply to the breast. The arterial supply to the breast is primarily derived from branches of the internal thoracic (mammary) artery, the intercostal arteries, and the lateral thoracic artery.

and serratus anterior muscles and send perforating branches through the chest wall musculature and out into the deep breast parenchyma.[27]

The internal thoracic artery is the dominant artery supplying the breast, and its branches supply the medial and central breast parenchyma. The lateral thoracic artery supplies the superolateral breast parenchyma. Branches of the subclavian and axillary arteries, including the thoracoacromial artery, the subscapular artery, and the thoracodorsal artery, often supply a portion of the superior breast parenchyma (Fig. 1.4).

Branches of the musculophrenic artery, a continuation of the internal thoracic artery, supply a variable portion of the inferior breast. The anterior and posterior intercostal arteries supply the deep central breast tissue by branches that perforate through chest wall muscles[28] (Fig. 1.4).

Superficial veins generally drain the center of the breast as well as the periphery and may have drainage connections to the contralateral breast. When superficial veins drain centrally, they

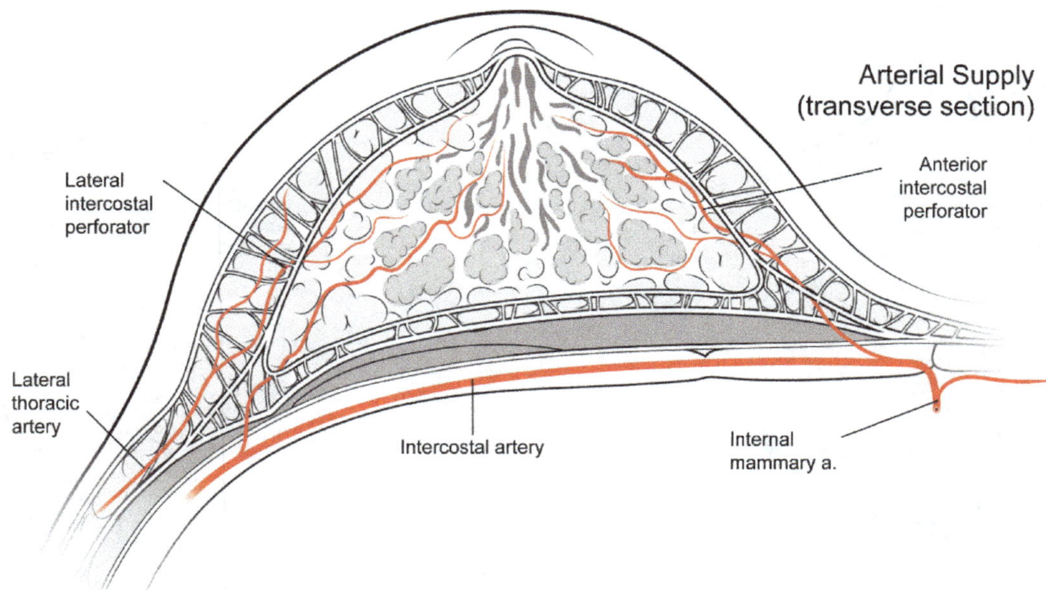

Figure 1.4. ■ **Arterial blood supply to the deep central breast tissue.** The anterior and posterior intercostal arteries supply the deep central breast tissue by branches that perforate through chest wall muscles.

usually converge on a peri-areolar circular network of veins (circulus venosus of Haller); from this venous plexus, venous blood is channeled into the internal thoracic veins medially and the lateral thoracic veins laterally.[28]

In the deep breast tissues, the venous anatomy of the breast parallels the arterial anatomy. Paired arterial and venous branches arise from the posterior intercostal, axillary, and internal thoracic (mammary) vascular pathways. Superficially, the venous anatomy is variable and does not accompany the arterial supply. Breast veins typically lack valves, and intramammary venous anastomoses are frequent.[29]

The existence of diverse, overlapping vascular networks explains why a variety of methods of breast reduction, based on various pedicles of different designs, can be performed safely, provided that the dissection is not too extensive, and the tissues are not twisted and sutured under tension[29] (Fig. 1.5).

Also, the advantage of nipple–areola pedicle de-epithelization makes sense in that it helps preserve the dermis and its circular superficial venous structures (Fig. 1.5).

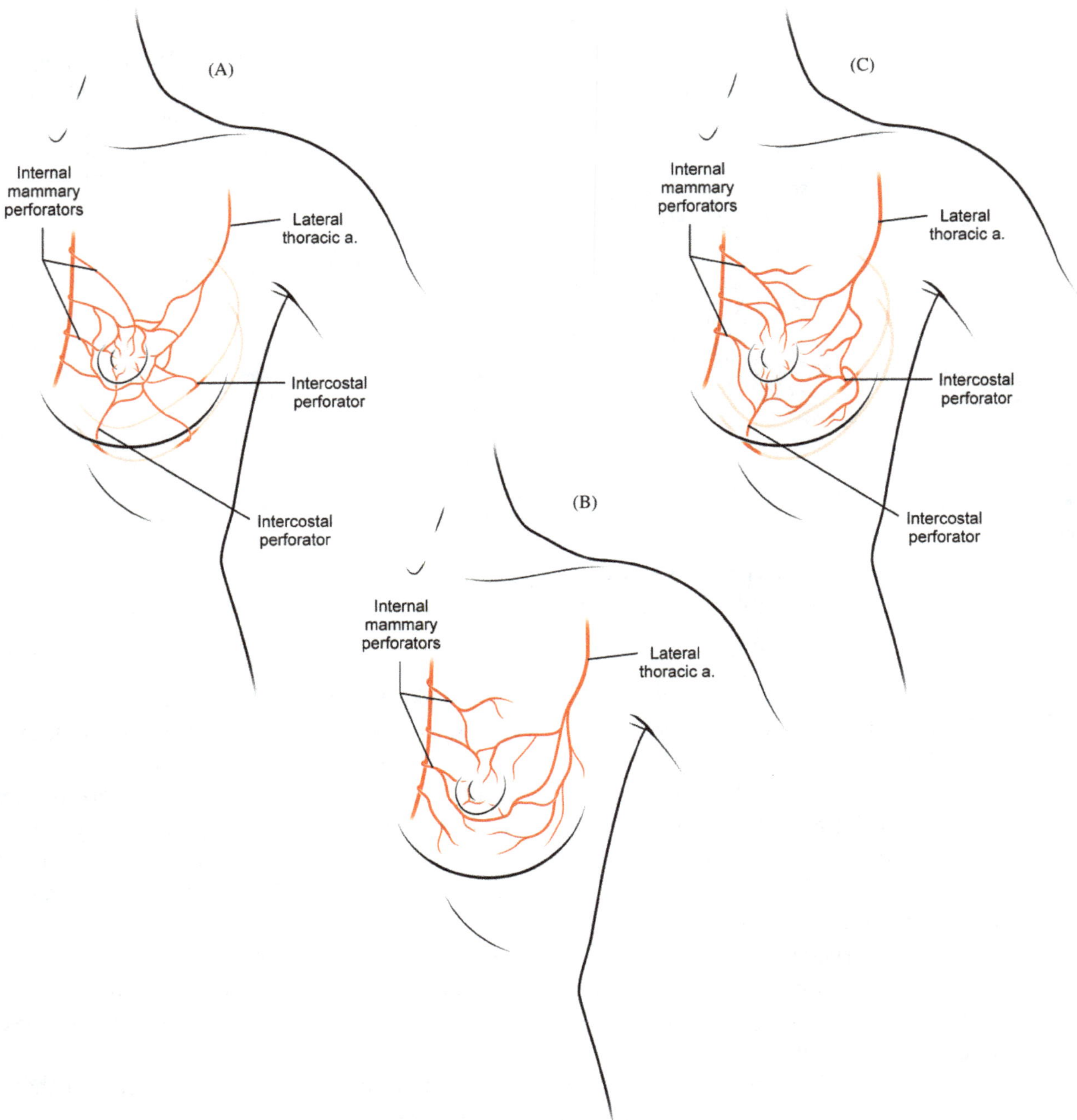

Figure 1.5. ■ Arterial blood supply to the breast. Note the variable arterial supply and collateralization. The illustration depicts three of the possible variations.

Innervation

The supraclavicular nerves innervate the superior portion of the breast from the third, fourth, and fifth branches of the cervical plexus. The anterior cutaneous branches of the second through seventh intercostal nerves supply the medial breast, both the skin and the gland. The nipple is primarily innervated by the branches of the fourth intercostal nerve, mainly the lateral branch. The lateral cutaneous branches of the other intercostal nerves travel subcutaneously to innervate the areola and the skin of the breast[30] (Figs. 1.6 and 1.7).

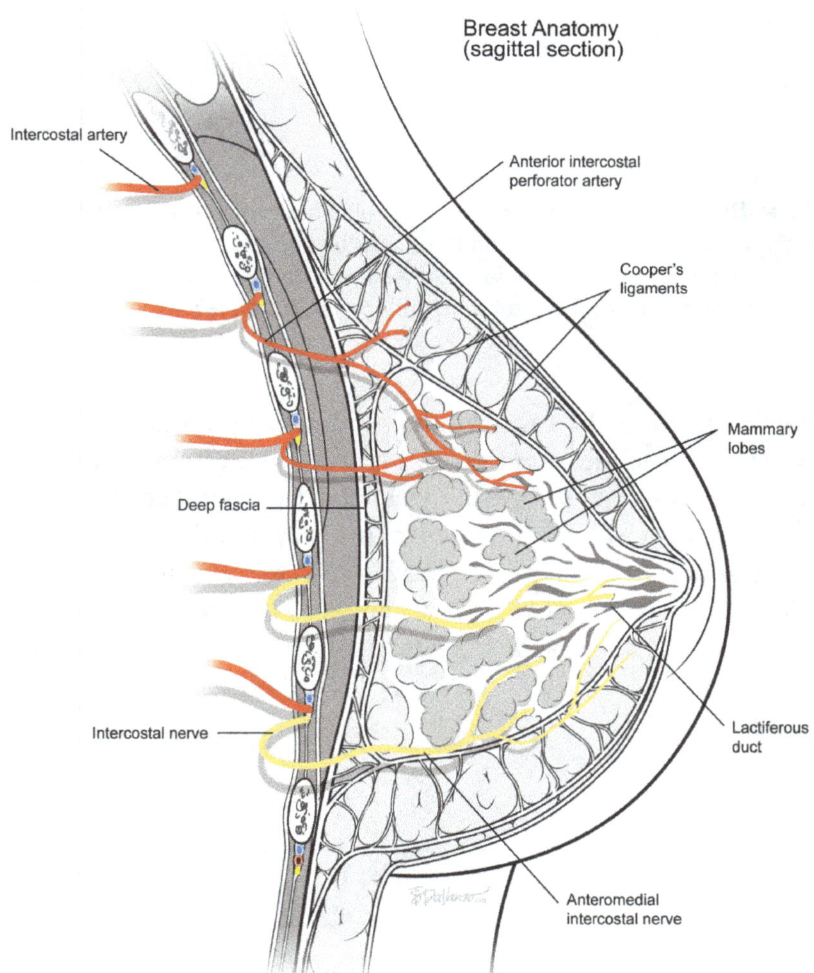

Figure 1.6. ■ Breast innervation. The nipple is primarily innervated by the branches of the fourth intercostal nerve, mainly the lateral branch. The lateral cutaneous branches of the other intercostal nerves travel subcutaneously to innervate the areola and the skin of the breast.

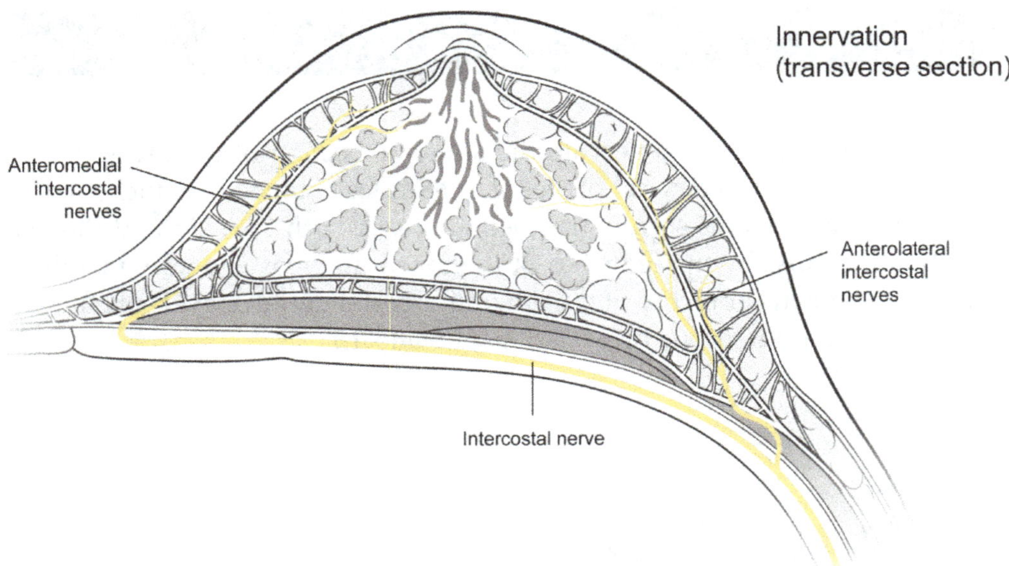

Figure 1.7. ■ Breast innervation. The lateral branch of the fourth intercostal nerve pierces the serratus anterior muscle at the midaxillary line and the fourth intercostal space. It then travels medially under the serratus anterior fascia and turns at a right angle at the level of the lateral border of the pectoralis major muscle, where it enters the posterior aspect of the mammary gland, approximately 1.5–2 cm from the edge of the gland.

The lateral branch of the fourth intercostal nerve pierces the serratus anterior muscle at the midaxillary line and the fourth intercostal space. It then travels medially under the serratus anterior fascia and turns at a right angle at the level of the lateral border of the pectoralis major muscle, where it enters the posterior aspect of the mammary gland, approximately 1.5–2 cm from the edge of the gland. The nerve maintains the same depth to the skin surface along its course toward the areola, until midway to the NAC. There its path becomes more superficial as it approaches the areola. At this point, it divides into five fasciculi that serve the nipple and the areola[31] (Fig. 1.6).

2

Multi-Level Mammaplasty

Fundamentals

Today a variety of breast-reduction operations, some new and some modifications of older techniques, combine parenchymal reshaping with the elevation of skin flaps, as is the case in peri-areolar, central, and inferior pedicle techniques.[32,33]

Despite the plethora of modifications and innovations, both the wise pattern and the vertical scar techniques fall short when applied to ptotic wide breasts.

In multi-level mammaplasty, the upper half of the gland is left attached to the skin and the areola on the de-epithelialized upper dermoglandular pedicle. The lower half of the breast, most of which is excised, is partially detached from both the skin (as in a subcutaneous mastectomy) and the chest wall, except for the breast pillars, which are sutured together below the new site of the areola. The nipple–areola complex (NAC) is based on a superior pedicle, which is broader in large breast hypertrophies. The superior pedicle can better withstand the forces of gravity, and if surgery is required in the future, recurrent ptotic tissue in the lower breast can be excised without the risk of cutting the former pedicle.

Tailoring the gland to shape the breast rather than relying on the skin to mold and maintain the breast shape is our preferred approach.

Multi-level mammaplasty places minimal tension sutures around the areola and the vertical scar. Breast shape relies on gland sutures. The excess skin on the lower pole is precisely excised and closed in a tension-free manner.

The following principles are the heart and soul of the Borenstein multi-level mammaplasty: (Homage to the "House of God" by Samuel Shem)

1. The breast ptosis comprises an inferior and LATERAL vector. The lateral vector has to be addressed.
2. A structure is only as reliable as its foundations.
3. A structure should be supported throughout its height.
4. The NAC should be finally placed after the breast mound has been structured.
5. Pre-surgical markings are only rough guides. Before any cut is made, the markings should be reassessed.

6. Eventually, the breast mound should be internally supported with no tension on the skin closure.
7. When considering hypertrophic or normal ptotic breasts, our goal should be to maximally narrow the breast mound because it tends to widen over time.

Surgical Principles of Multi-level Mammaplasty

Multi-level mammaplasty is a technique that relies on a superior pedicle for the NAC and involves a lower central breast reduction, glandular shaping, and suturing. Less scarring is involved than with the inverted T incision but more than with the peri-areolar technique. This scar may, at times, extend beyond the IMF onto the chest wall. However, if the scar matures favorably, it will fade over time and be partly obscured by the breast (Fig. 2.1).

Upper pole

The planned NAC is based on a superior pedicle. Therefore, the upper pole of the breast remains attached to the skin and the areola on a partially de-epithelialized upper dermoglandular pedicle (Fig. 2.2).

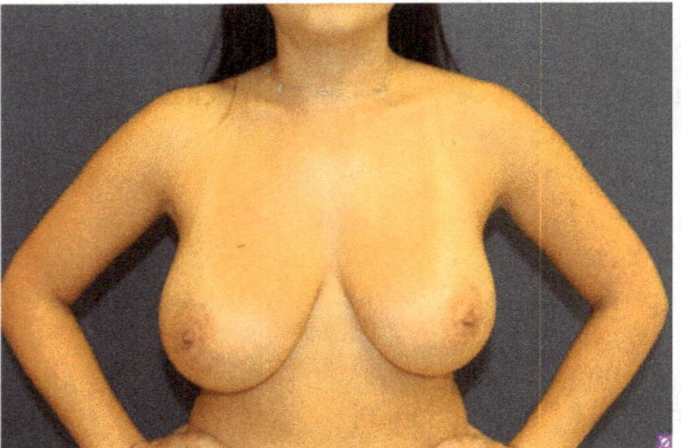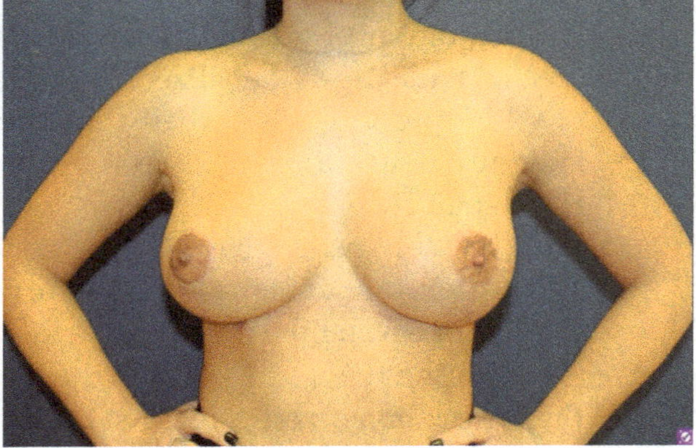

Figure 2.1. ■ **Multi-level mammaplasty.** Before (left) and 1 year after (right) the surgery. Note the right breast scar extending to the chest wall.

Inferior pole

Most of the excision is done in the lower half of the breast. Once the excision is completed, the remaining breast tissue will serve as "pillars," situated below the upper pole. However, this term is misleading because these breast tissue "pillars" cannot support the breast mound on their own. Instead, the "pillars" serve as a starting point from which we may shape the breast and recreate the support that was lost over time, or due to fluctuation in breast mass, or as a result of our dissection (Fig. 2.3).

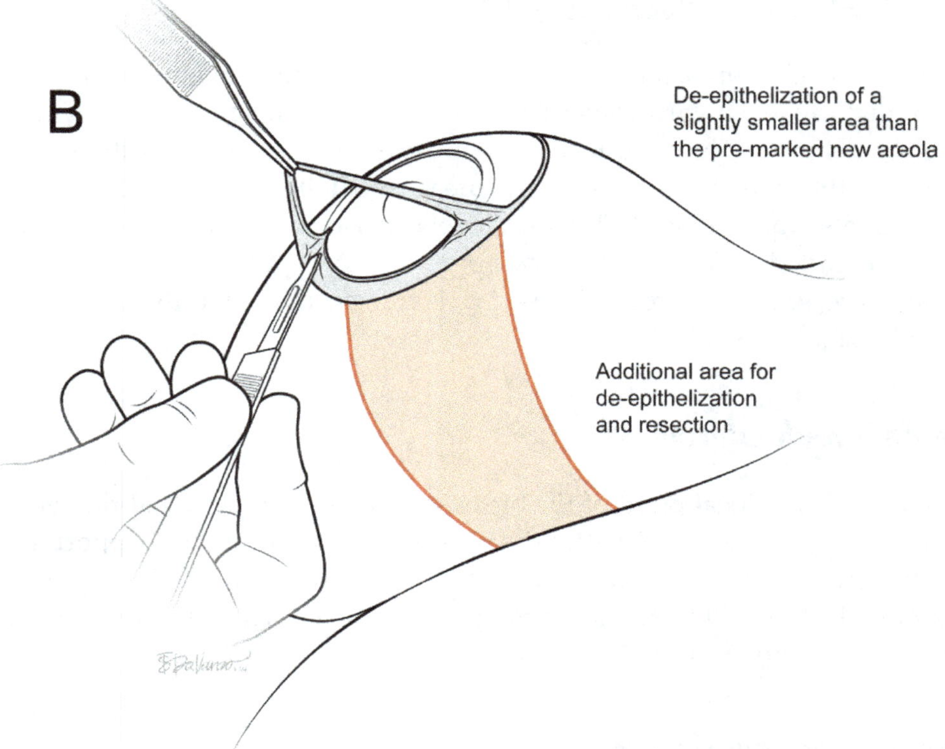

Figure 2.2. ■ **Upper pole.** Note the partially de-epithelialized upper dermoglandular pedicle.

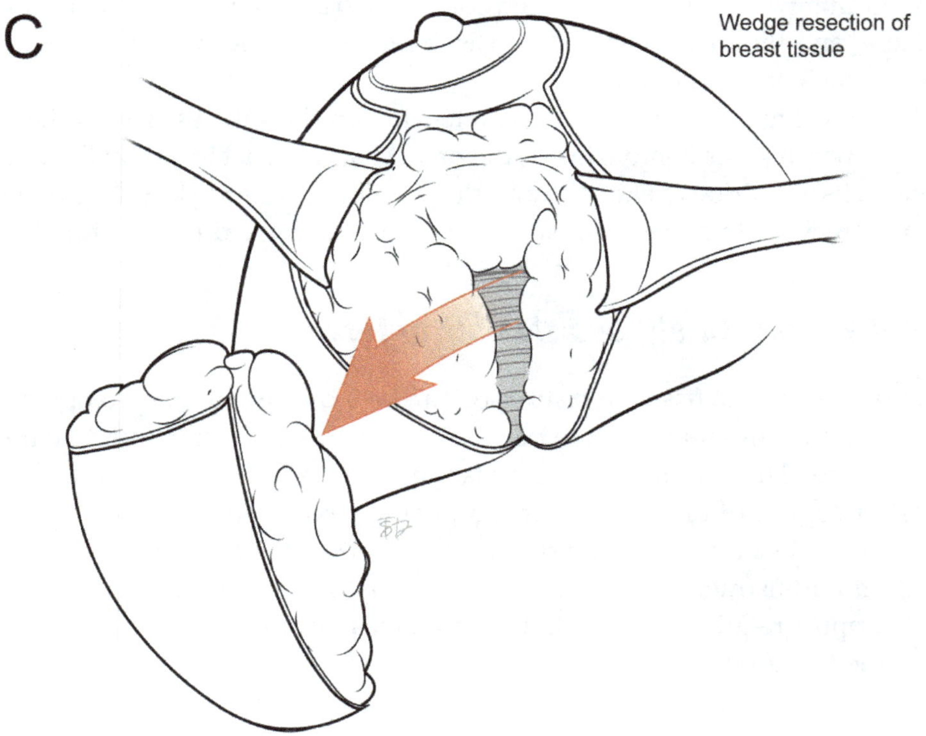

Figure 2.3. ■ **Lower pole.** Note that the excised tissue can be extended under the NAC as needed.

Multi-level breast mound support

The multi-level approach refers to the breast when the patient is in the supine position, from the pectoralis fascia outward toward the skin. We can imagine the restructuring of the breast as building a house. The base level of the breast is the closest to the chest wall. The base-level sutures gather the lateral pole of the breast medially to the pectoralis fascia. The second level approximates the "pillars." The third level consists of repeated absorbable sutures on the superficially denuded surface of the now approximated "pillars" to tightly pack and invaginate the tissue in breast circumference. These levels transform the width of the breast into projection and upper pole fullness (Fig. 2.4).

Nipple–areola placement

The nipple is the focal point of the breast and should be placed at the most projected part.

This can only be verified after the multi-level breast mound support has been completed and the patient seated. Then an external suture is put to mark the bottom of the future areola. De-epithelization of the areola opening is completed achieving the proper tension-free circular shape, and insetting of the NAC is accomplished.

Tension-free skin closure

Skin elasticity varies with the individual and is influenced by the amount of tension exerted on the skin. That is why techniques that rely on the skin to act as a "brassiere" for the breast have disappointing results. Though less tension leads to a flat and ptotic breast, more tension improves the shape, and the likelihood of necrosis, infection, dehiscence, and unattractive scars increases in conditions with higher tension.

Multi-level mammaplasty places no tension on the sutures around the areola or on the vertical suture because the contouring of the breast has been achieved by the multi-layered sutures of the breast tissue. Prior to skin closure, the previously raised skin flaps on either side of the "pillars" are precisely trimmed so that the "rest" approximated just waiting to be sutured (Fig. 2.5).

Symmetry, scars, safety, and stability of results

The amount of breast tissue to be excised can be indicated by the pre-operative markings. On the other hand, the amount of skin to be excised is determined only after the breast mound has been reconstructed. The combination of a planned volume adjustment and "free-hand" closure enables better control of final nipple–areola opening, placement, and tension-free skin closure.[34]

The multi-level breast mound support serves a triple purpose. First, it facilitates gradual control and adjustment of the lateral breast contour and breast width. Second, it recreates the fascial support required to maintain stable breast shape. Third, it translates it to projection and upper pole fullness.

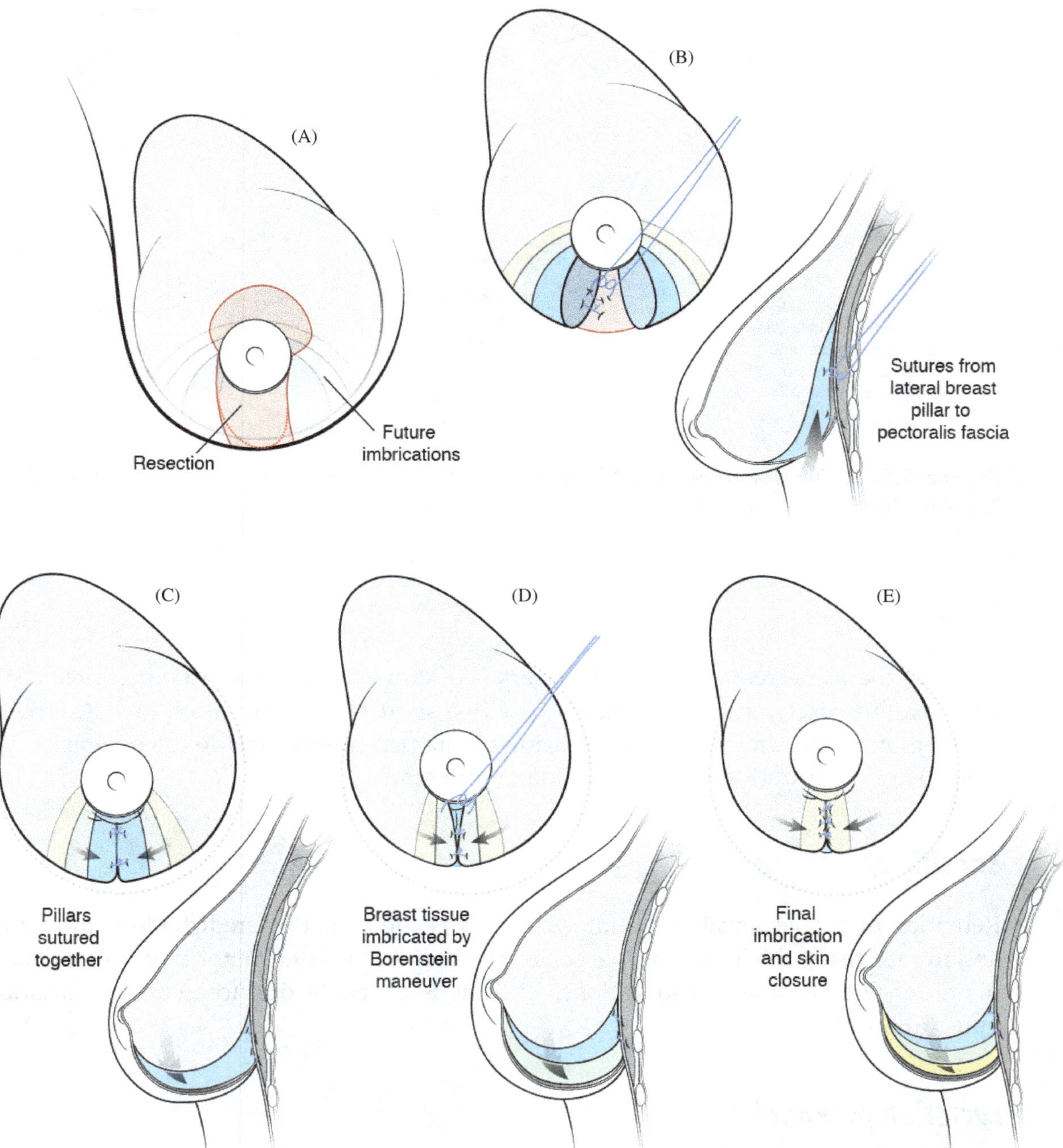

Figure 2.4. ■ **The multi-level mammaplasty from bird's eye view.** Note the translation of width to projection. A. Illustration showing the skin and central portion excision in red and the three levels of breast tissue to be imbricated. B. Breast following central portion excision and medial sutures to the pectoralis fascia. Note the initial effect of narrowing the breast on anterior posterior (AP) view and the outward (projection) upward vectors on lateral view. C. First level of the Borenstein maneuver. Note the narrowing of the breast on AP and outward (projection) upward vectors on lateral view. D. Second level of Borenstein maneuver. E. Third level of the maneuver to close over with the breast skin in a tension-free manner.

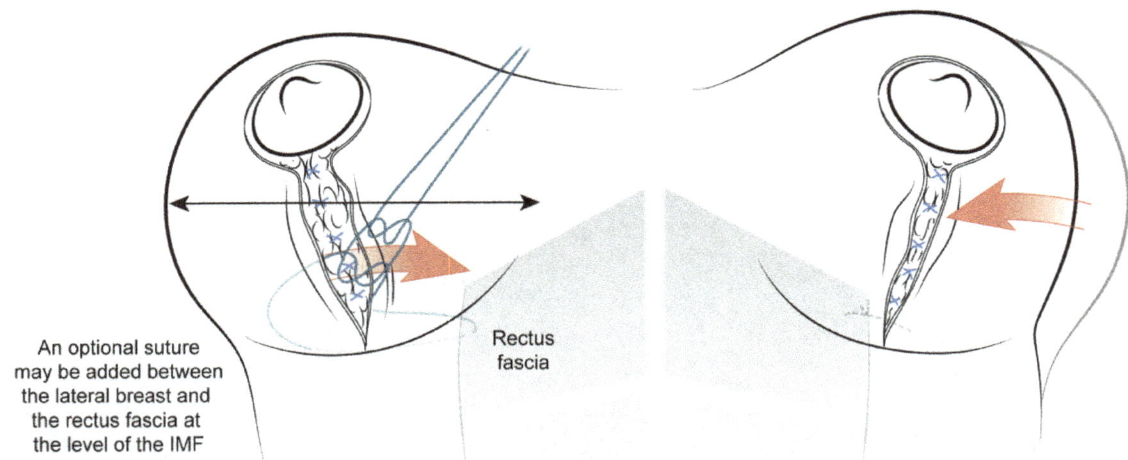

Figure 2.5. ■ **Tension-free skin closure.** Note the way the skin flaps are approximated with no tension, following the multi-level sutures and precise skin trimming.

Scars

Limiting the scars created by breast surgery is of utmost importance to our patients. With multi-level mammaplasty, the peri-areolar scar with a short vertical extension obviates the need for a submammary scar and reduces the tension on the peri-areolar scar. Reduced tension is the principal factor contributing to the formation of thin scars.

Sensitivity

Retention of nipple sensitivity and erectability is somewhat unpredictable with any technique, and in rare cases, the loss of nipple sensitivity may occur after minor breast reductions, even in the absence of healing complications.[35–40] This is probably due to anatomic variations in the innervation.[41,42]

Lactation potential

Theoretically, lactation should not be hindered.[43] Depending on the extent of resection, some sub-nipple ducts and glandular tissue are preserved. Strömbeck demonstrated that lactiferous ducts interrupted by surgery partially reunite post-operatively, possibly as a result of hormonal stimulation during pregnancy. This study explains why lactation is not impaired even by techniques that cut the gland close to the areola.[44]

Adaptability

Multi-level mammaplasty can be used to reduce very large breasts and to tighten and lift ptotic ones. Because the markings are individualized for each patient, and the final de-epithelization, extension, and skin excision are done after the necessary breast mound support and shape are achieved, the technique can be adapted to all breast sizes and shapes.

Multi-level mammaplasty aims to achieve safe and reproducible results, volume and contour correction, improvement of symmetry, limited and favorable scarring, preservation of sensation, and limited effect on lactation potential.

Another not less important goal of our method is to become an easy-to-learn technique, allowing secondary operations, markings, and adjustments to all types of breasts.

In the following chapters, the implementation of the multi-level mammaplasty principles in breast reduction (Chapter 4), combined breast implant explantation and mastopexy (Chapter 5), and combined breast augmentation and mastopexy (Chapter 6) is described. Materials regarding post-operative breast support and complications are presented in Chapters 7 and 8, respectively. Scars are separately discussed in Chapter 9.

3

Patient Consultation and Evaluation

Before treatment is planned, a woman's motivations as well as her desires for breast contour merit scrutiny. Patient expectations need to be fully explored to ensure that they can be met. It is critical to determine the desired breast size — too big or too small is not acceptable.[45] The surgical plan must provide the patient with the optimal breast shape and size with minimal scars.

Consultation, Motivations, and Indications

When a patient seeks consultation about breast surgery, the surgeon must first determine why she is seeking treatment at this particular period in her life and assess her expectations.[45,46] For adolescents, it is often clear that they seek treatment as soon as their parents can be persuaded. Often, they are accompanied by their mother, who may ask if their daughters are too young for such an operation. Once both mother and daughter are reassured, the decision is straightforward, and the operation is scheduled to coincide with the school holidays. Adolescents are typically concerned about the reduced breast size but do not often ask about postoperative pain, scars, or nipple sensitivity.

Younger patients with breast hypertrophy have high expectations for an excellent result. However, they typically have firm skin that is predisposed to scarring despite the reduction technique used. Efforts to limit scar length are of particular importance for this group of younger women.

Diverse factors motivate older patients with large breasts.[47] They may have delayed seeking treatment until their children have grown, their financial status has improved, or their husband's resistance has been overcome. Surprisingly, they are usually not sexually driven. Instead, they seek reduction because of the discomfort caused by the excess breast weight, the limitations on sports activities, imposed by their large breasts, and the difficulty in finding clothing that adequately accommodates the size of their breasts.[45] If they even mention sexual concerns, it is to inquire about post-operative nipple sensitivity or to express their companions' concerns about not wanting their breasts to be too small.[48] They are concerned about post-operative shape, volume, symmetry, and short scars, but they usually have reasonable expectations.[48]

The least demanding patients are older women who have suffered from their deformity for years and are delighted at the prospect of relief from the physical discomfort associated with their heavy breasts. In older patients, the resulting scars tend to be thinner and less prone to hypertrophy.[49]

In our experience, patients who seek correction of ptosis are very different from those who want a breast reduction. The former group is the most demanding, and they often unrealistically expect that the operation can recapture the youthful firmness and elevation that characterized their breasts earlier in life. The unavoidable scars and the presence of striae make this an unattainable goal. Most of these women have little understanding of the role skin elasticity plays in the stability of the result. Because of the poor quality and inelasticity of their tissues, patients with ptotic breasts may be prone to recurrent ptosis, which occurs post-operatively, regardless of the surgical technique chosen.[50]

In light of the above, before surgical correction is planned, a discussion between surgeon and patient, about what can realistically be achieved through surgery, is critical. Again, it is essential to understand the patient's motivation in seeking surgical correction at this point in her life. With a woman who has experienced breast involution after childbearing and breastfeeding, and plans no further children, this decision is usually well thought out. She often has the support of her husband, has realistic expectations, and accepts the fact that the scars take approximately 1 year to fade, and that the quality of the result may deteriorate over time.[51]

On the other hand, a patient who has experienced an abrupt and traumatic change in her personal life, such as a divorce or the death of a loved one, may expect immediate and dramatic improvements. Such women frequently request mastopexy as well as body contouring. Some take sufficient time to weigh their decisions; others impulsively decide to have the operation. These patients are not always psychologically prepared for the post-operative consequences and may struggle to endure them, mainly if complications occur. They typically lack patience in accepting that the result will evolve, and they are critical of minimal problems with scars and shape.[52] Usually, such patients do not disclose that they are having personal problems. The surgeon can avoid a potentially troublesome situation by paying attention to the patient's attitudes during the consultation.

Patients with unrealistic expectations should be evaluated with the greatest of care. They may have previously met with another surgeon, who proposed placing a breast implant rather than performing a mastopexy. Although implant placement is an easy solution, this approach is simplistic and does not adequately address the problem.[49] It is always challenging to explain to such patients that they need a total reshaping of the breasts, which inevitably involves some scarring. It is a common misconception that the ptosis stems from the loss of breast volume, and therefore can be adequately corrected by the placement of an implant. Such patients fail to consider that the skin of their breast has stretched as a result of pregnancy, lactation, or aging processes and requires resection.

Some patients with large, ptotic breasts request a mastopexy without reduction. We have to warn them that post-operative recurrent ptosis is expected, because large breasts are more likely to succumb to the forces of gravity, especially in women who have already experienced ptosis.[49] After a frank discussion, these women can make a decision based on a realistic expectation for the result of the surgery.

Patients with large breasts who request a reduction so significant that their breast size would then not be compatible with their body size pose a dilemma. We believe that the patients should always have the final say about their body. However, we do not think that just because an operation can be performed, it automatically should be. Therefore, if we feel uncomfortable operating, we will communicate this to our patients, and, perhaps, decide not to operate.

Some women decide to undergo breast surgery to please a companion, not because they desire it for themselves. We always try to discourage such women from having surgery, because we feel that their reasons are not sound and that they may regret this decision later.

Contraindications to breast reshaping surgery are uncommon, and most patients are appropriate candidates for the operation. However, some women believe that their quite healthy breasts are abnormal in comparison to the large firm breasts of women depicted in the movies, on television shows, and in fashion magazines. These patients, who request a mastopexy for a minor problem, would fail to sufficiently benefit from an operation to justify the resultant scars. Surgeons who consult these women need to invest time and patience to reassure them that their feelings of inadequacy are ill-founded and that any surgical procedure has limitations. Indeed, it is more difficult and time-consuming to say "no" than "yes" to a patient who requests an operation. These patients are often perfectionists, who perceive their body as ill-balanced, making it almost impossible to convince them otherwise. In such cases, we sometimes choose to inform them that though they will eventually find a surgeon willing to operate on them, they might regret undergoing surgery, since the scars are permanent.

Patients with local skin problems, such as submammary maceration or mycotic infection, can be considered as candidates once these conditions have resolved. General health problems such as hypertension, diabetes, and lung diseases can now be better controlled and are not in themselves considered contraindications.

We do not routinely perform esthetic breast surgery on patients with a BMI over 32 kg/m^2. Overweight adolescents are advised to diet, and the desired operation is offered as the reward for their effort. Obese mature women have more to gain by primarily addressing their weight problem and then seeking breast surgery. We have found that operating on patients with a BMI over 32 kg/m^2 leads to considerably higher complication rates. On the other hand, patients that comply and lose the excess weight before surgery also tend to attend follow-up visits and, generally, have more realistic expectations.

Medical History and Physical Examination

A detailed personal and family history of breast diseases is obtained from every patient. A thorough physical examination for any mass in the breasts and axillary regions is mandatory. A preoperative mammogram is required for women with a personal or family history of breast cancer or breast disease and all patients over the age of 35 years.

The first consideration during the consultation is the patient's habitus and we determine the satisfactory breast volume and shape to her body. *Then we consider the sternal notch to inframammary fold (IMF) distance. This is often overlooked, but in our experience, it is vital to inform the patient that the breast will eventually settle within this distance.* Next, we assess the ptosis of the breast, namely, how low the nipple–areola complex (NAC) descends under the IMF. This helps to plan the distance which we will raise the NAC to.

In our method, the breast width in relation to the patient's chest wall is of great importance. The larger the discrepancy between the patient's chest wall and breast, the better the results will be, compared to alternative techniques.

Hi-profile implants — we find that our patients prefer the immediate esthetic appearance achieved by using hi-profile implants. Our patients describe the dramatic step-off achieved by using these implants as having better upper pole fullness without significant disturbance to the narrow breast we aim for. Nevertheless, we acknowledge that implant choice is a very subjective decision and would stress that any implant can be selected by using the described methods with great success.

Volume — The implant volume is chosen according to the patient's breast width and the previously chosen profile.

Informing the Patient

The details of the operation should be carefully explained to the patient. In particular, she should be told what can be expected from the operation, where the scars will be placed, the degree of the proposed reduction in terms of brassiere cup size, and how long it will take until her breasts attain their final shape. This information is especially important to convey to patients undergoing multi-level breast mammaplasty, which results in an initial upward displacement of the breasts.

The surgeon should not underestimate the importance of scar appearance to the patient. Patients who have a breast reduction or mastopexies are equally concerned with resulting scars, breast shape, and volume. Prominent scars negate the benefits achieved by breast reshaping.

It is important to describe the position of the scars to the patient and to inform her of how long it will take for them to smooth out and fade. We explain that the areola is the most visible part of the breast, and that the appearance of the peri-areolar scar is thus one of our primary concerns. We also explain that to create the multi-level structure, we "invaginate" breast tissue in the central aspect of the breast under the vertical scar, which may lead to temporary wrinkles. These wrinkles disappear in a few weeks in most women, and by 3 months in women with very large breasts. Patients readily agree that this temporary puckering is an acceptable price to pay for the limited scars and the desired structure of the breasts.

The surgeon, familiar with the anatomy and physiology of healing, naturally has more patience with the healing process than the patient, who is anxious to see the outcome of the operation and who is not as understanding of the time it may take for the scars to fade and for the breast form to mature.

Unless complications occur requiring special treatment, the surgeon's role after the operation is to reassure the patient and to urge her to follow his recommendations. Excellent communication skills are essential at this stage for calming the patient's fears and educating her about the anticipated post-operative course and the expected short- and long-term evolution of the results.

We insist on visually demonstrating to the patients the expected result using similar-looking breasts from former real-life cases. Specifically, we use the illustrations, presented in Fig. 3.1, to

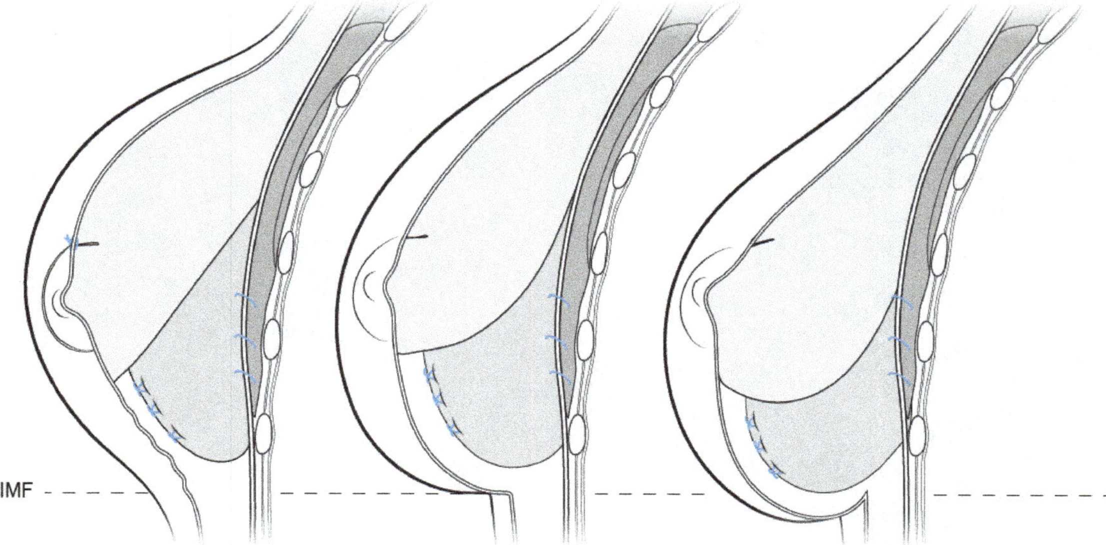

Figure 3.1. ■ **Natural progression of breast descent after surgery**. Note the way the breast mound descends at 1 month (middle) and 3 months (right) after the multi-level mammaplasty. Eventually, the lower pole lies below the IMF.

demonstrate to the patients the natural course of breast shape formation and encourage them to memorize it.

The operations described in this book usually cannot deliver a "perfect result." Therefore, proper management of expectations via an open and frank discussion is a crucial factor in building and maintaining a healthy and happy patient population.

4

Multi-Level Breast Reduction

According to the American Society of Plastic Surgeons (ASPS) national plastic surgery statistics, 43,591 breast reduction procedures were performed during 2018,[53] implementing a variety of available surgical options, modifications, and innovations. So why invent a new procedure?

Twenty years ago, the senior author (AB) came to an understanding that the common conception, according to which the breast reduction methods should mainly address the correction of the inferior ptosis, was misguided. Along the years of experience, it became clear that the ptotic breast has a significant lateral vector to the ptosis as well. Therefore, correcting only the inferior vector may lead to wide breasts with a lack of projection.

Another problem was the feeling that most existing methods attempted to reconstruct a breast without proper foundations, despite the trivial notion that given no proper support, high constructs cannot be built. Finally, a large number of breast reduction patients presented with wide breasts still posing a significant challenge for most of the available reduction methods, which typically did little to address this width and left a disproportionate breast shape. The Borenstein maneuver was created as a way to trade-off between width and projection by aiming at taking the laterally displaced breast in, toward the cleavage line, and creating a projection.

Surgical Technique and Rationale

Marking and de-epithelization

The breast is marked as in a vertical scar reduction procedure (Figs. 4.1 & 4.2).

After marking, preparing, and draping the supine patient, de-epithelization of an area, slightly smaller than the pre-marked new areola, is carried out. This is because in our method we

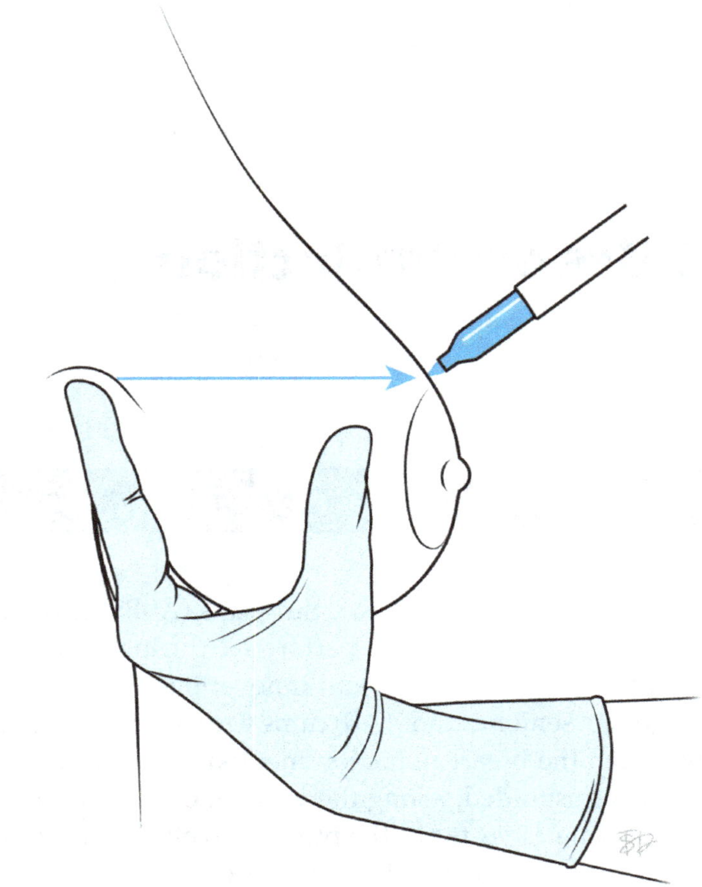

Figure 4.1. ■ Marking the future nipple–areola complex position. Note the positioning in the expected most projected part of the breast.

find it hard to predict the exact amount of skin to be excised. As a rule of thumb, a deflated breast will have more skin excised than a full and firm breast. Final de-epithelization is completed upon the breast mound formation (Fig. 4.3).

Lateral support

Next, the central wedge resection skin incision is made with a scalpel followed by electrocautery dissection down to the pectoralis fascia (Fig. 4.4).

Next, the undermining of the breast tissue above the pectoralis fascia is extended, as would be done for a sub-glandular implant pocket (Fig. 4.5).

The lateral support is created by 1–3 absorbable vicryl 0 (Johnson & Johnson Medical N.V., Belgium) sutures, which should be put between the lateral breast tissue and

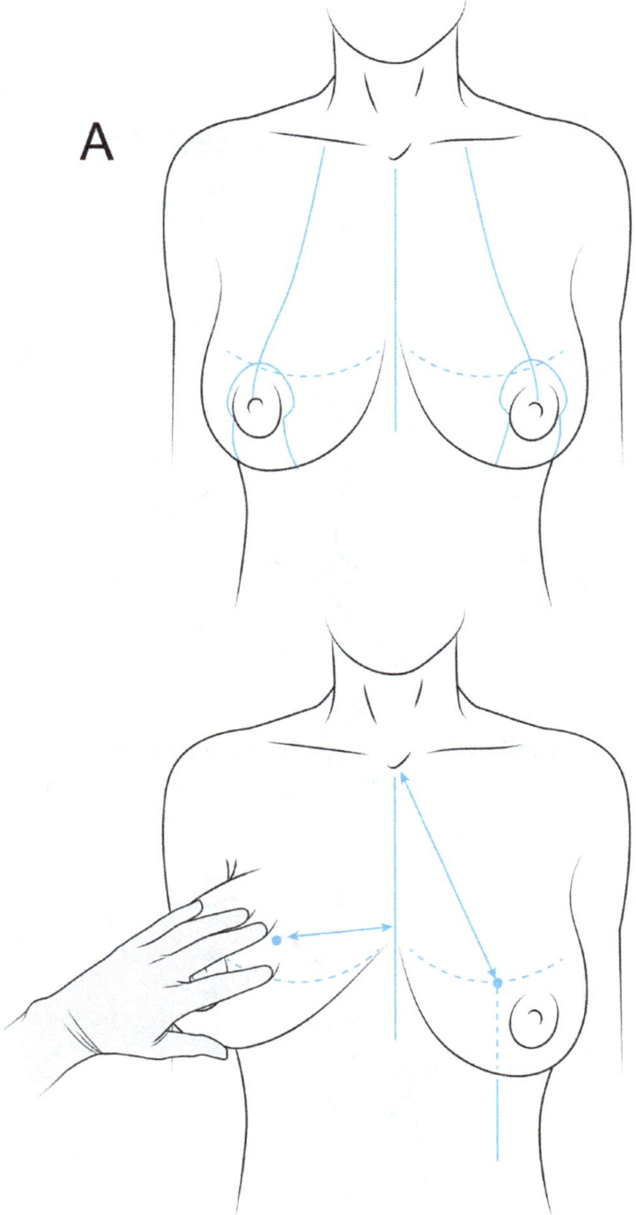

Figure 4.2. ■ **Marking the expected de-epithelization and excision borders.** Note the Lassus maneuver moving the breast from side to side to determine the safe limits of tissue resection.

the pectoralis fascia, just medial to the breast meridian at 30 degrees upward angle. **Importantly,** the former sutures cannot be tied down before their effect on the lateral breast slope is visualized. The previous step can be repeated more superficially with 2–3 sutures in larger breasts (Fig. 4.6).

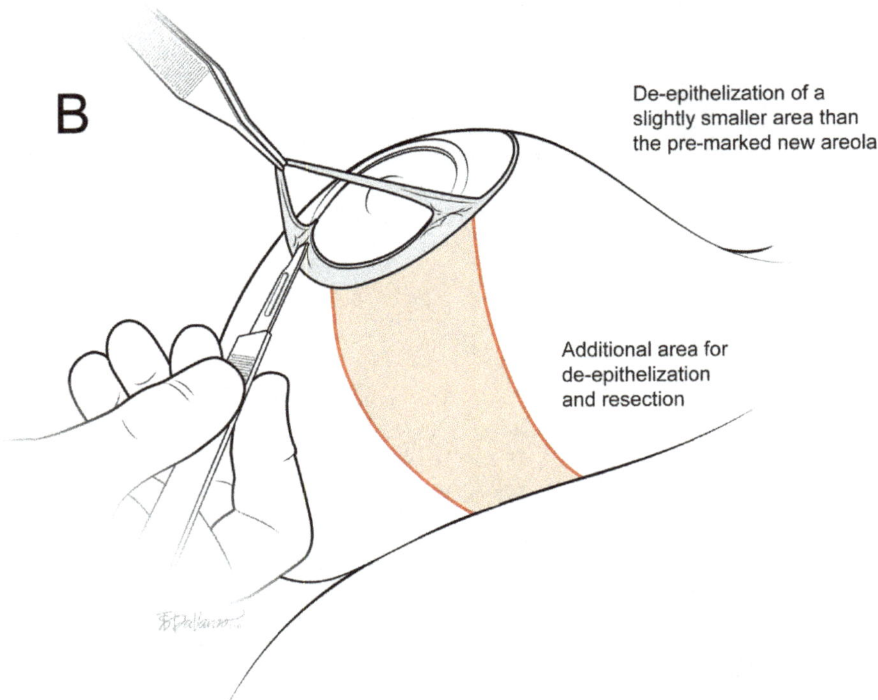

Figure 4.3. ■ De-epithelization. Note the conservative de-epithelization that will be completed after the final recreation of the breast mound support using the multi-level mammaplasty technique.

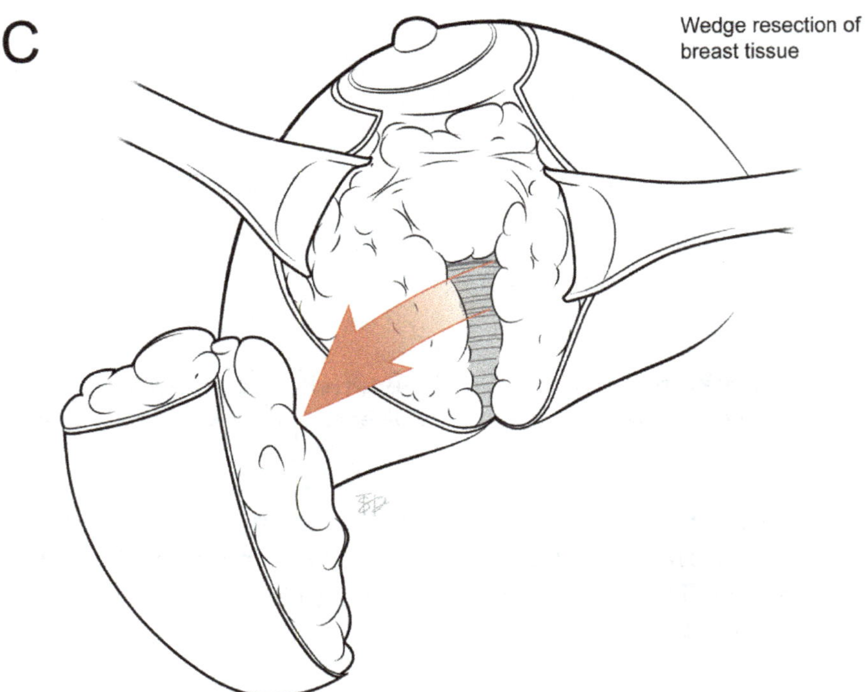

Figure 4.4. ■ Lower pole tissue resection. Note that the actual resection can be extended superiorly under the NAC if needed.

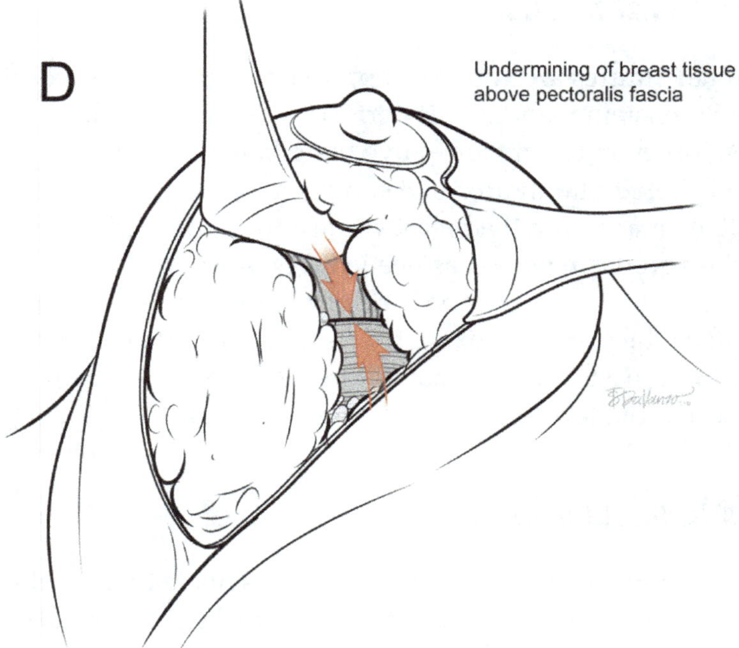

Figure 4.5. ■ **Undermining of the breast tissue.** Undermining of the breast tissue above the pectoralis fascia is extended, as would be done for a sub-glandular implant pocket.

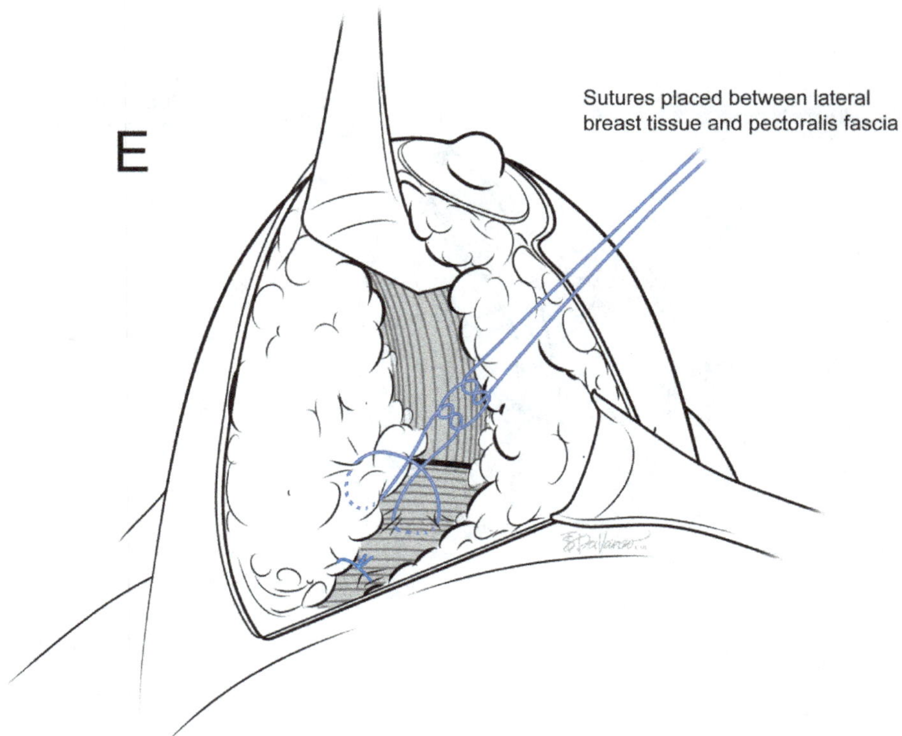

Figure 4.6. ■ **Lateral sutures.** The lateral support is created by 1–3 absorbable vicryl 0 sutures.

Shaping the breast mound

One to two pillar sutures are added to approximate the pillars loosely (Fig. 4.7).

Next, the Borenstein maneuver is performed — two thin dermal flaps, similar to facelift skin flaps, are developed on either side above the pillars (Fig. 4.8).

Two to four horizontal figures of 8 sutures are put at the freshly exposed breast tissue edges above the pillars, narrowing the breast while adding projection (Fig. 4.9).

The previous step is repeated as needed (Fig. 4.10).

When the expected breast shape is achieved, the excess thin skin strips are cut, and the tension-free dermal edges are approximated using an absorbable intradermal suture (Fig. 4.11).

In very wide breasts, an optional suture may be added between the lateral breast and the pre-rectus fascia at the level of the inframammary fold (IMF).

Nipple–areola complex insetting

The patient is then seated, and an external suture is made to mark the bottom of the future areola. A dyed cookie cutter is placed over the nipple–areola complex (NAC) and surrounding skin, to mark the new areola opening. De-epithelization of the areola opening is made and insetting of the NAC is completed (Figs. 4.12 & 4.13).

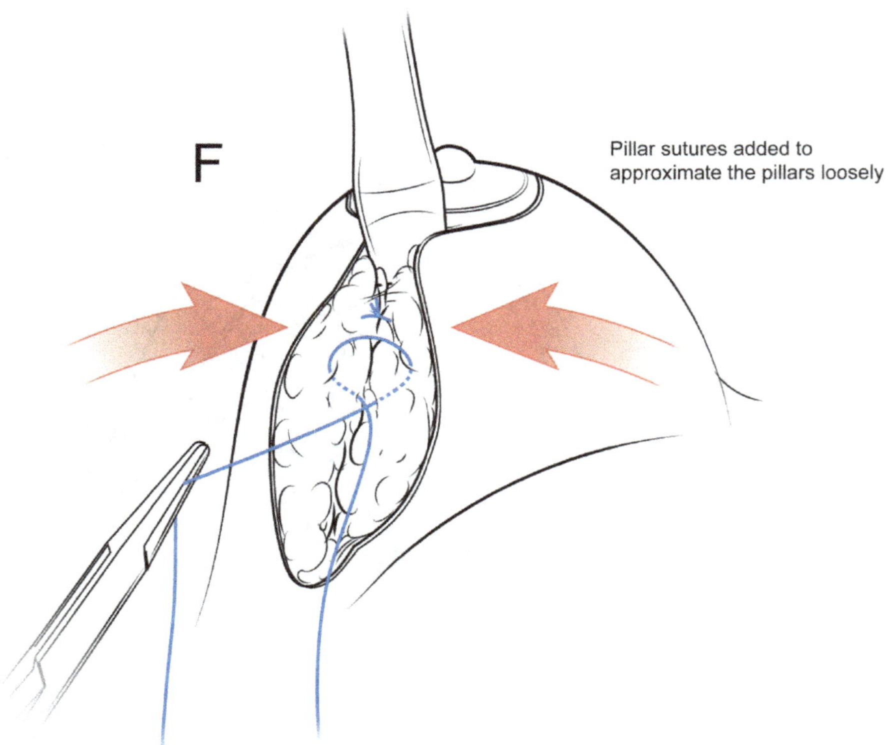

Figure 4.7. ■ Pillar sutures. 1–2 pillar sutures are added to approximate the pillars loosely.

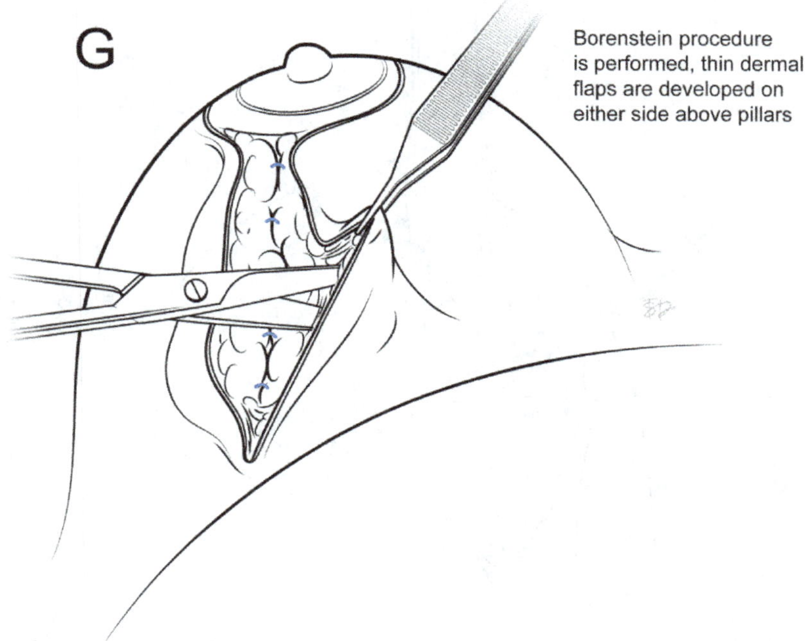

Figure 4.8. ■ **Raising the skin flaps.** We prefer using scissors for this step.

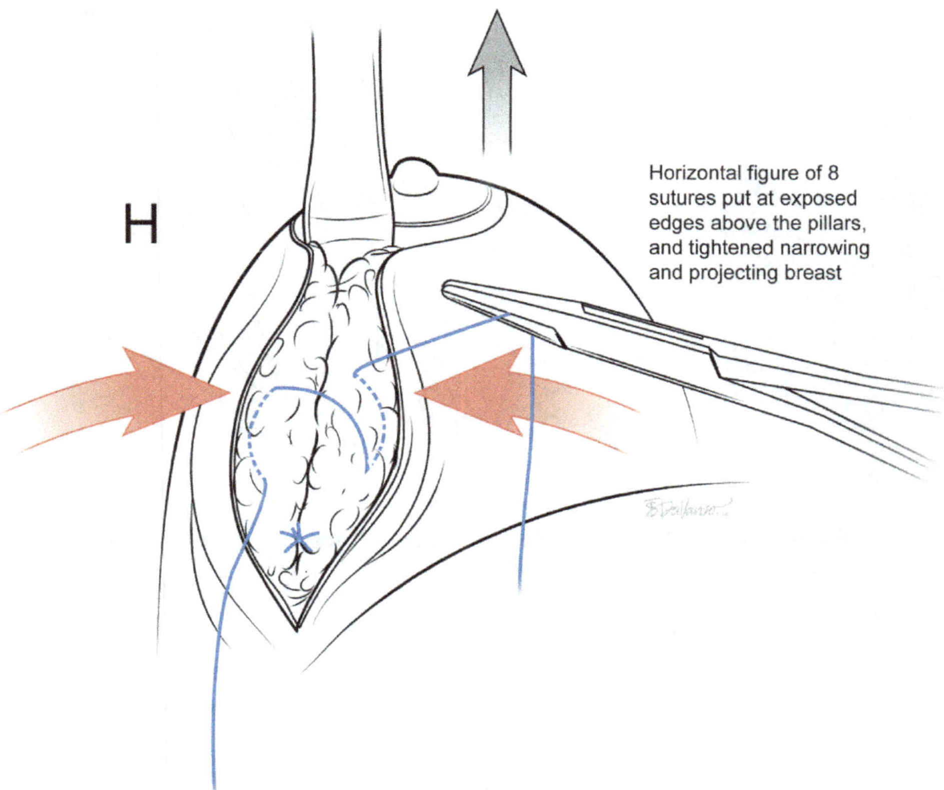

Figure 4.9. ■ **A single figure of 8 sutures.** These sutures effectively imbricate the breast tissue, narrowing the breast while adding projection.

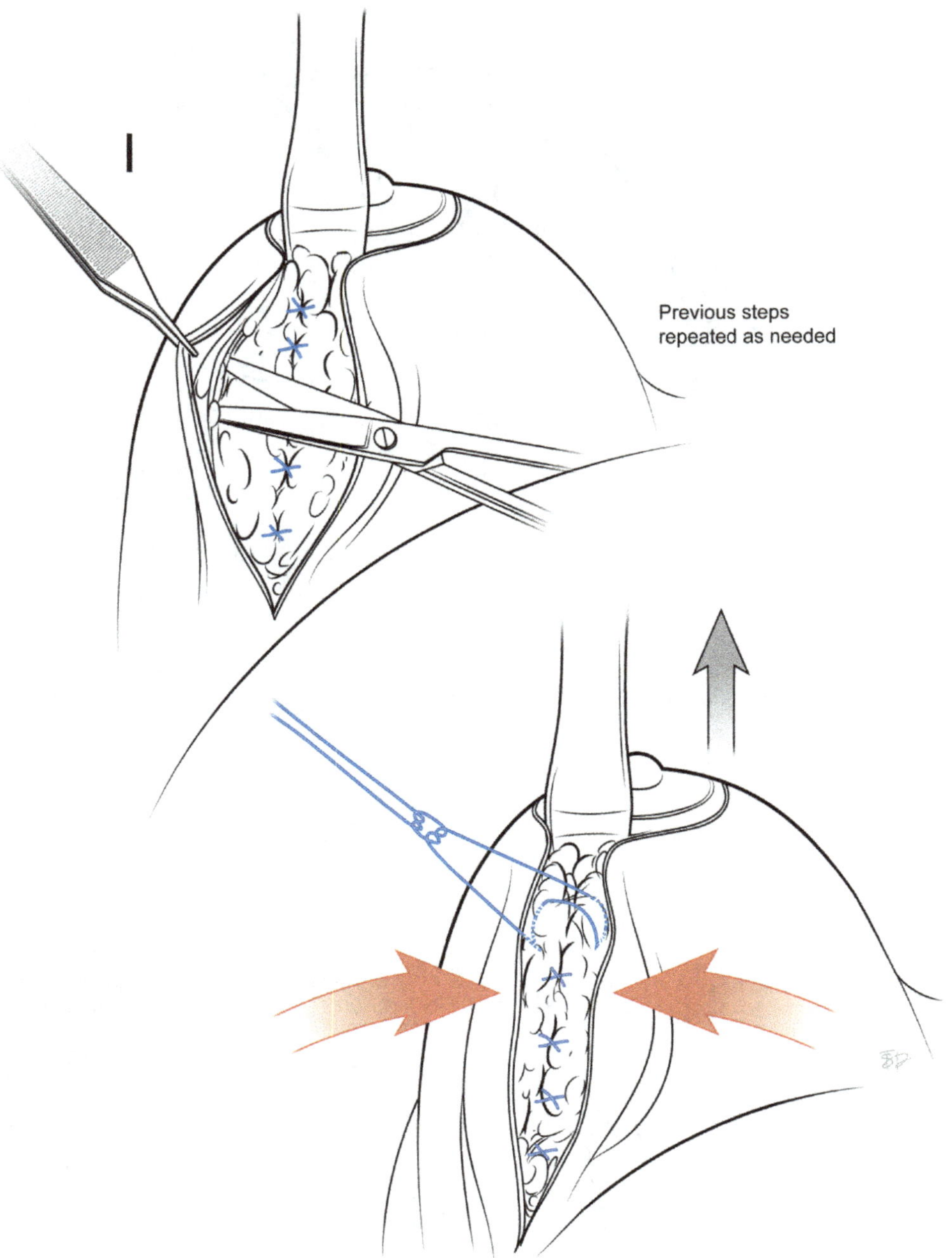

Figure 4.10. ■ **Repeating the Borenstein maneuver.**

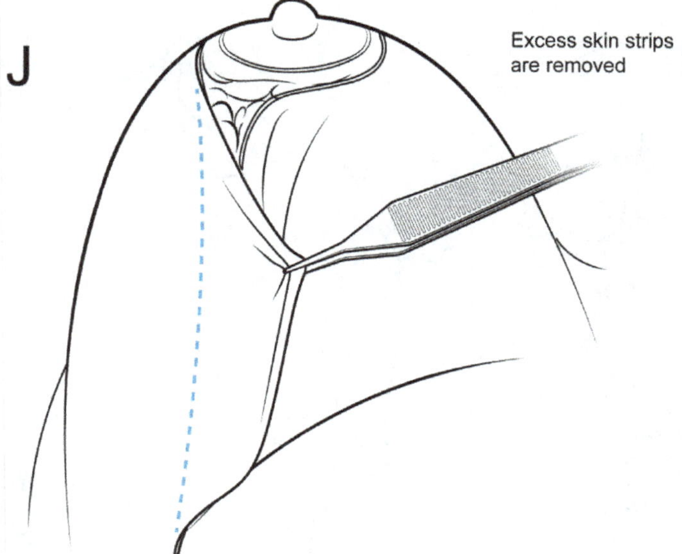

Figure 4.11. ■ **Precise trimming of the skin.** For a tension-free closure.

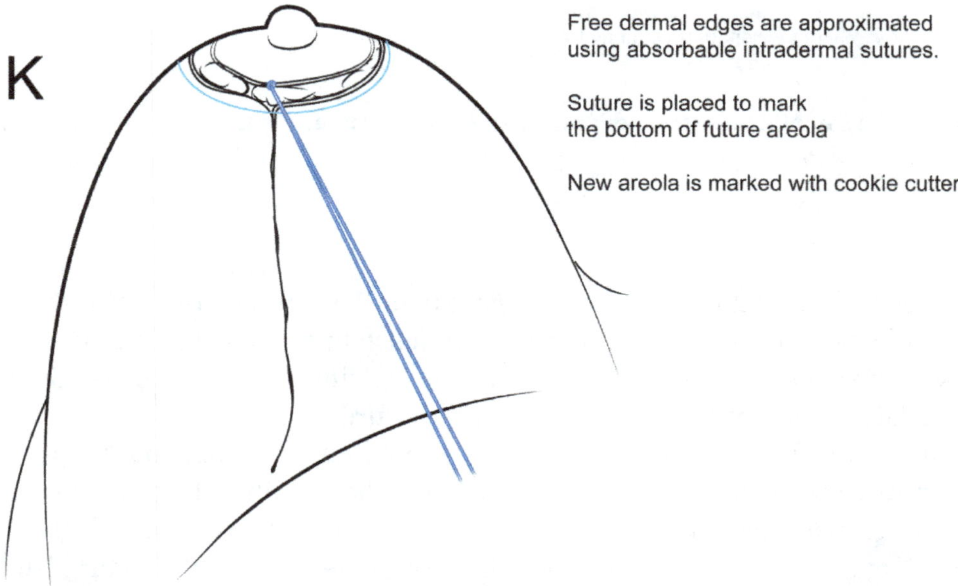

Figure 4.12. ■ **Nipple-areola complex final de-epithelization.** This is the final step, after the recreation of the breast mound.

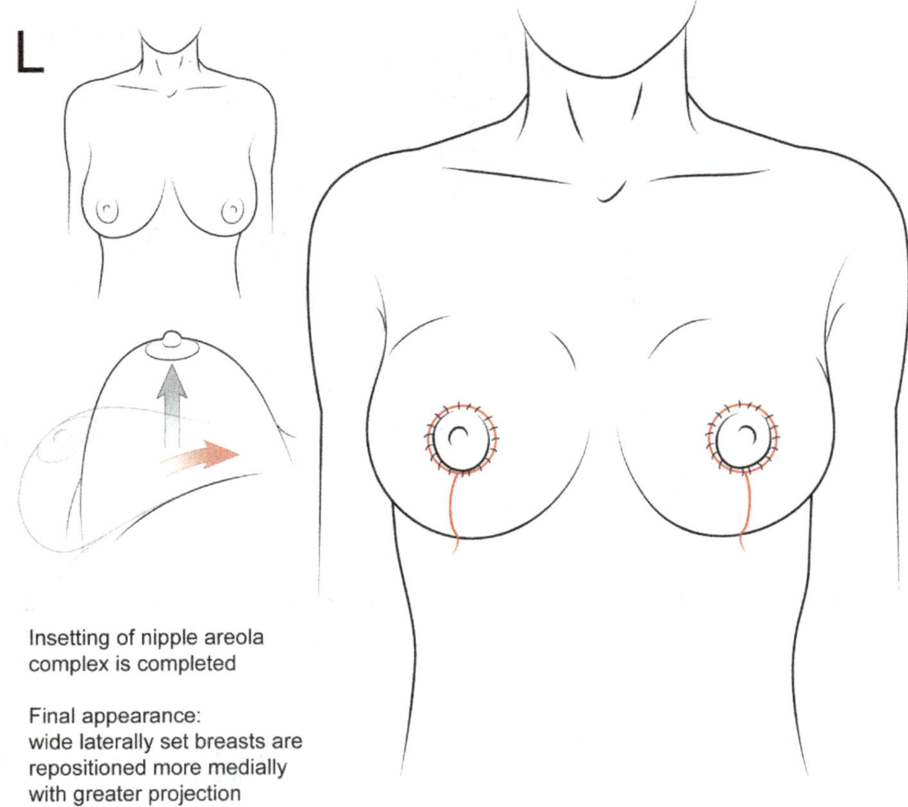

Figure 4.13. ■ Nipple-areola complex (NAC) placement. Note how the change in projection may change the final location of the NAC.

When the method was developed, more than 15 years ago, the main concern was the survival of the thin skin flaps created during the Borenstein maneuver. This was partially solved by a stepwise progression during the maneuver, creating at each step 1–1.5-cm wide flaps to be excised later to accommodate a tension-free closure.

Still, up to 20% rate of minor dehiscence continued to trouble our patients. The development of the paper bra postsurgical dressing technique has finally solved this problem (Fig. 4.14).

Initially, we typically removed the paper bra at postoperative day (POD) 14. This practice reduced minor dehiscence rates but did not solve the problem completely. Postponing the removal of the paper bra to POD 21 eliminated minor dehiscence occurrence almost completely. Routine assessments for examining the NAC and the dressing for any secretion or discharge are carried out at POD 1, POD 7, and POD 21.

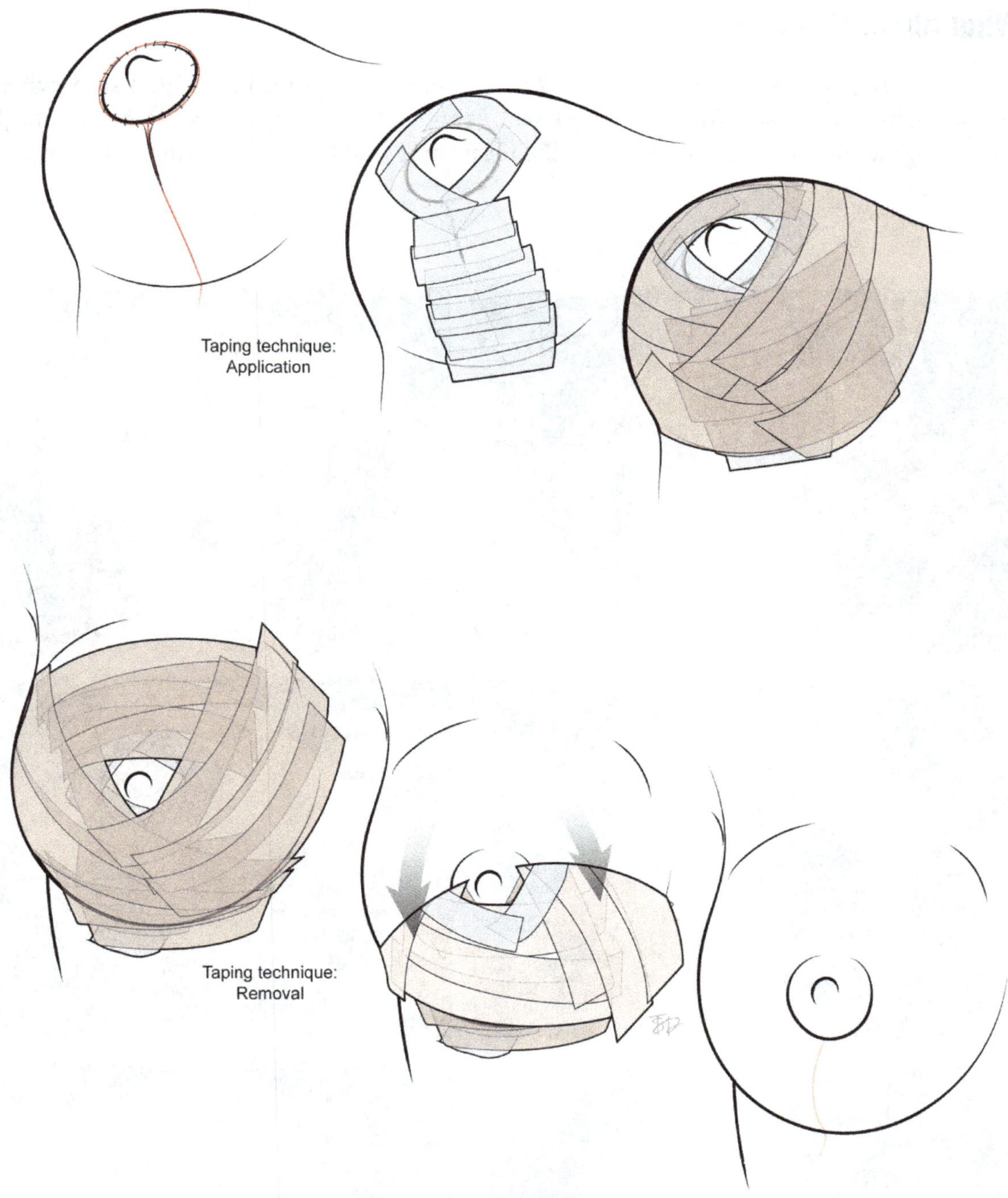

Figure 4.14. ■ **Paper bra postsurgical dressing technique.** Note the added external support of the dressing.

What About Mastopexy?

A mastopexy is performed the same way as reduction except for one added step, where all the breast tissues are raised from the chest wall, similar to creating a pocket for a sub-glandular breast augmentation. This step releases the tissue and enables restructuring of the smaller breast (Fig. 4.15).

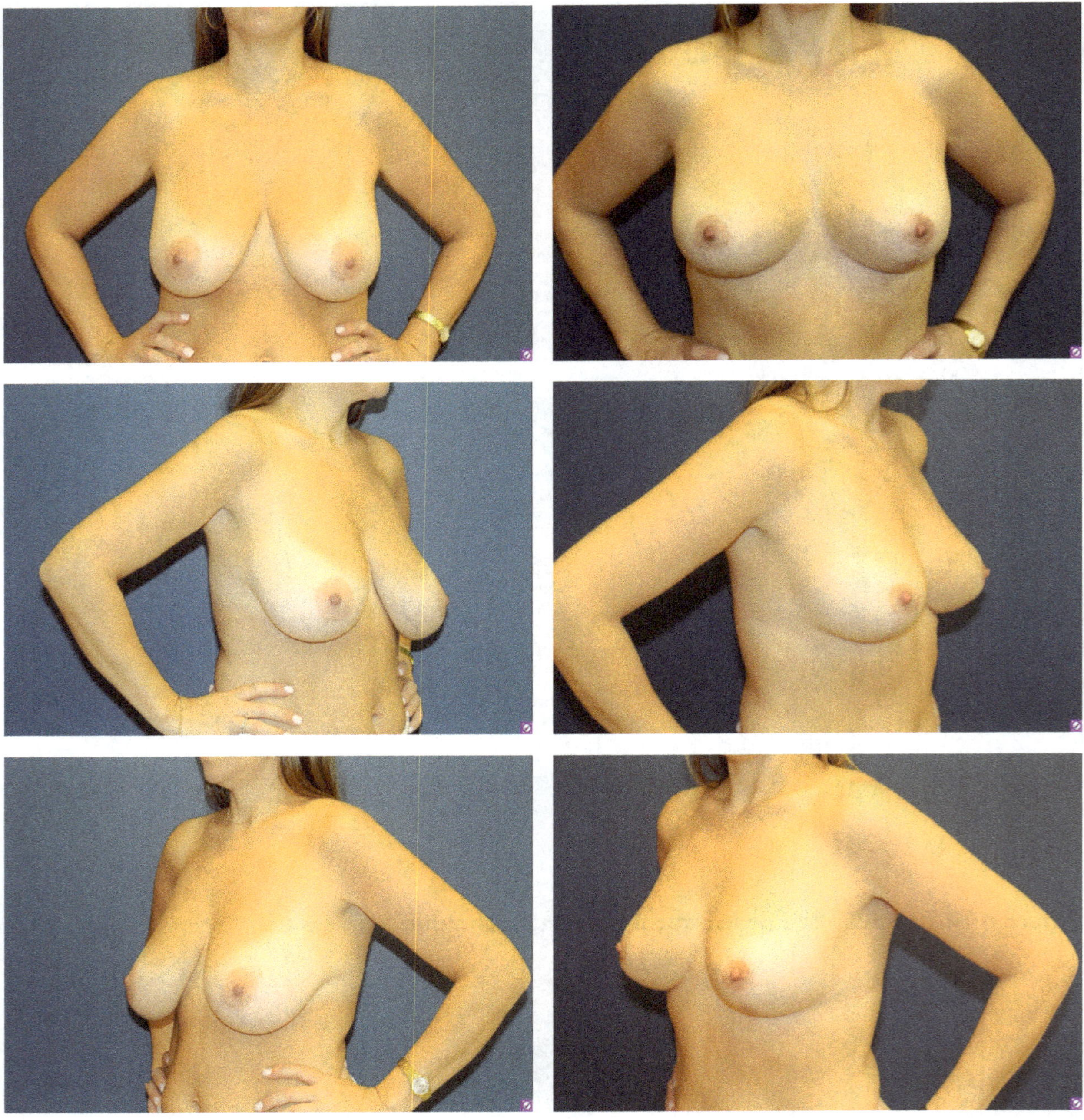

Figure 4.15. ■ Treatment of large ptotic breast. Before (left) and 1 year after (right) surgery. Note the tailored treatment of the ptotic breast.

Concluding Thoughts

Most of the cited methods debulk the breast tissue, taking care to preserve the NAC, and pack it all in with a tailored skin "brassiere." Some authors have attempted to address the shaping of the central portion of the breast via pillar suture, or by suspending the pedicle in attempts to augment the upper pole. However, essentially, such "construction" of the reduced breast is comparable to building a house from the roof down, sometimes without even addressing its foundations. With the idea of shaping the breast mound bottom up, the senior author (AB) developed the Borenstein Breast Reduction (BB-R) technique.

The BB-R technique targets three previously undertreated characteristics of the overly large breast: 1. Lateral displacement of the breast. 2. Horizontal breast access (wide breasts). 3. Projection (Figs. 4.16 & 4.17).

The technique follows the rational markings of a vertical scar breast reduction. Initial skin and breast tissue excision are limited to the vertical limbs, set by the "Lasuss maneuver." The breast mound foundation is set by lateral to medial absorbable sutures, bringing in the unruly lateral breast tissue and fixing it to the pectoralis fascia. Building upon the new breast mound foundation, the "Borenstein maneuver" is applied in a stepwise manner to incrementally expose superficial breast tissue and snugly imbricate it over the approximated pillars. This step is critical, in that it translates the horizontal breast access to projection. Moreover, the stepwise execution of the maneuver facilitates an intuitive shaping of the breast, similar to a child building a sandcastle on the beach. Finally, this method adapts the tissue laxity to the final skin excision.

The figures of 8 sutures support the vertical arrangement of the collected tissue. When the wanted projection is achieved, the skin flaps, raised above the now invaginated breast tissue, are excised to facilitate tension-free closure, and at this point, the bottom of the areola is marked with a suture. The final placement of the areola, reminiscent of Pitanguy's original description, helps to inset what will be the focal point of the breast in a best-controlled manner[4] per the aesthetic relations of the breast.[34]

In our published series of 338 cases, complication rates are comparable or lower than previously published series.[2–8,32,33,54] The relatively high rate of superficial dehiscence (68 patients, 20%) could be explained by our strict reporting criteria, which included every patient who was prescribed any local treatment during the follow-up visits, typically, the areas of superficial dehiscence located at the junction between the bottom part of the areola and the vertical scar near the IMF. Their size ranged from a pinpoint opening, marked by a delicate crust, to an opening of the scar with part of the intradermal Monocryl suture knot showing. None of our cases needed any form of re-closure in office or otherwise. The three (0.8%) patients, taken back to revision surgery in our series, suffered from hematomas. We do not routinely use drains or lipoaspirate in breast reduction surgery and they are highly suspicious of any "bruising" or irregular swelling after surgery.

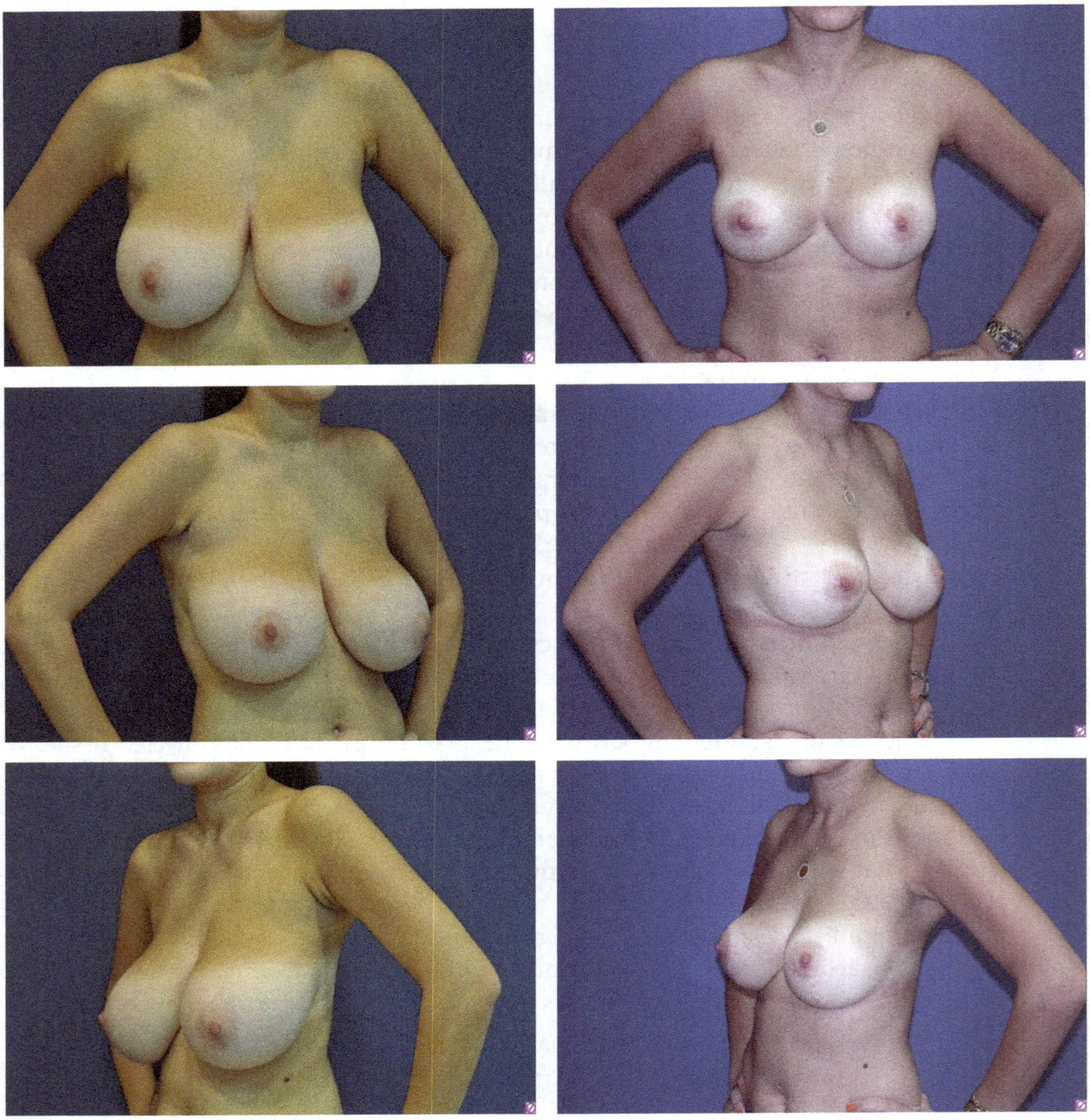

Figure 4.16. ■ Overly large breast reduction. Before (left) and 5 years after (right) surgery. Note the tailored treatment of key elements.

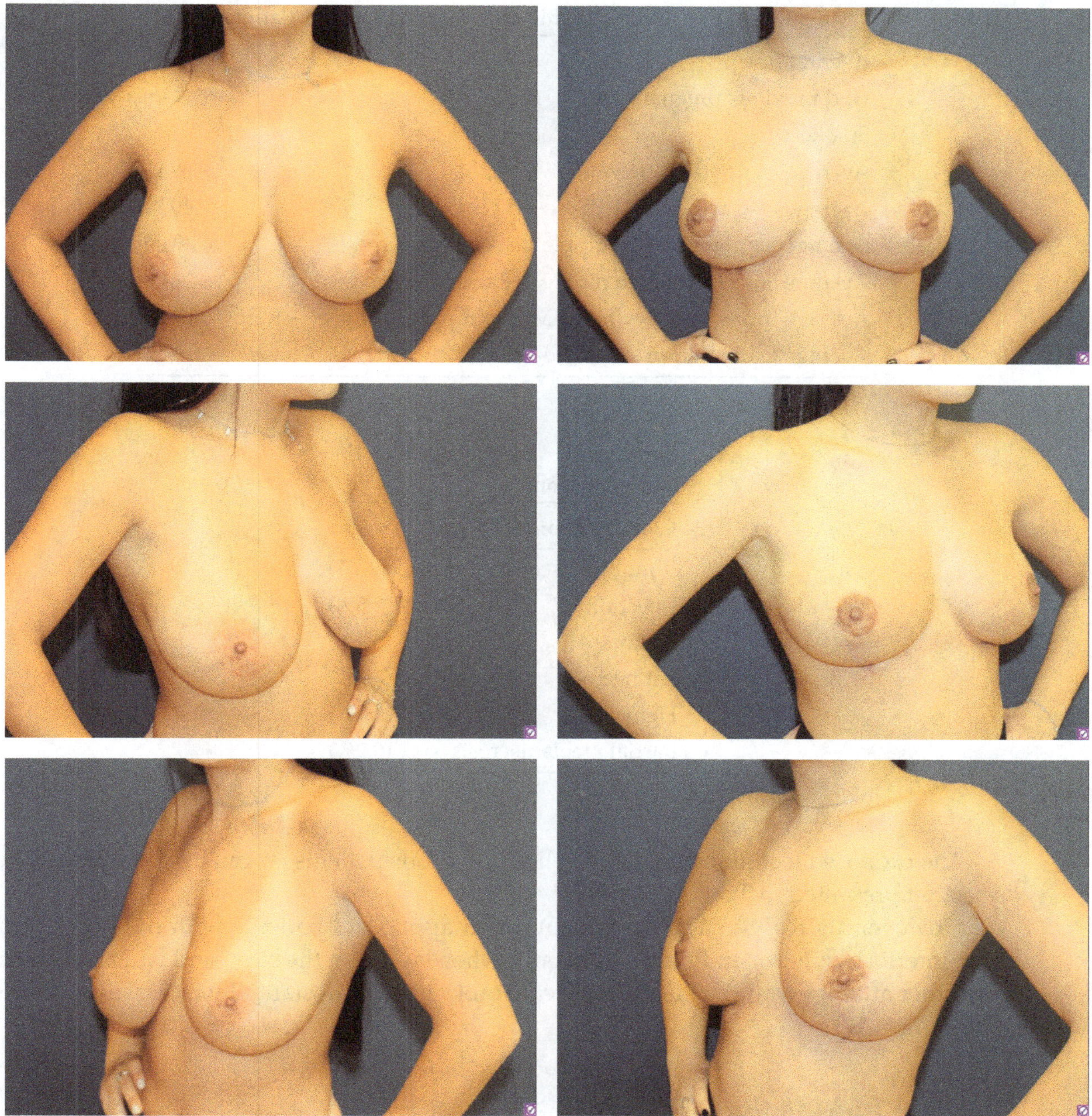

Figure 4.17. ■ **Treatment of large and asymmetric breasts.** Treatment before (left) and 1 year after (right) surgery. Note the challenging correction of asymmetry while maintaining projection and proportion of the recreated breasts.

Table 4.1. Demographic and Surgical Data of Patients

Average age	34
Had previous pregnancies	146
Smokers	51
Average resected tissue weight — Right	395 g
Average resected tissue weight — Left	400 g
Average Sternal notch to nipple distance — Right	29 cm
Average Sternal notch to nipple distance — Left	29 cm
Average inframammary fold (IMF) to nipple distance — Right	13 cm
Average IMF to nipple distance—Left	13 cm

Table 4.2. Summary of the Complications

Complication	$n = 99$
Minor dehiscence	68 (20%)
Infection	12 (3.5%)
Seroma	11 (3.2%)
Fat necrosis	4 (1.2%)
Hematoma	3 (0.8%)
Partial areola necrosis	1 (0.2%)

The proposed technique may be applied to various patients, as can be observed by the varied selection presented in Tables 4.1 and 4.2.

However, its real strength is evident when applied to patients with medium-sized ptotic, both inferiorly, when standing, and laterally, when laying on the back, and wide breasts, in which any other attempt would either fail to create projection or substantially increase the complication rates (Fig. 4.17).

Tips and Tricks to the Technique

1. Markings and de-epithelization are similar to any superior breast lift.
2. Following the central wedge resection, undermining of the breast tissue above the pectoralis fascia enables the reorganization of the breast mound foundation. It helps to imagine the implant the surgeon would have picked for the patient considering her chest width and habitus.
3. Medialization of the laterally displaced breast tissue using lateral sutures controls the lateral vector of breast ptosis and creates the foundation for a pleasing new lateral slope and narrow base for the rest of the breast.

4. Layered closure of the vertical scar converts breast width to projection, aids the final NAC positioning, and reduces tension from final intradermal skin sutures.
5. NAC opening final de-epithelization and placement is done as the last step when the breast mound is reconstructed, and its position can be verified in a 3D manner.
6. Liposuction is a powerful tool when addressing the tail of the breast or overweight patients with considerable lateral rolls. We also use it for final touchups of the entire inferior pole.

Limitations

There are several limitations associated with the BB-R technique. First, the lateral sutures, though essential for building the foundation of the breast mound, may lead to dimpling in the lateral breast. This is difficult to treat if not identified during placement, and often a compromise on breast shape should be made if dimpling is to be released. Second, the vertical scar may, at times, lengthen to the abdominal wall. We appreciate the logic of Lejour and Hall-Findley's approach and the use of liposuction as an adjunct to breast reduction procedures.[41] However, we do not routinely perform liposuction during a breast reduction, so we cannot remark on its merits; perhaps this may help in the final shaping of the lower pole of the breast and facilitate further skin tightening in selected patients. In patients with poor skin quality conversion to limited inverted T scar may be prudent. In our experience, scars extending beyond the IMF to the superior abdominal wall are well tolerated by our patients, as long as they have been appropriately informed, and the scar is hidden by the inferior pole of the breast when their hands rest alongside their body.

Summary

The BB-R technique is a safe, reproducible surgical option, which addresses some of the previously undertreated problems of oversized breast — wide, laterally displaced, and unruly breast tissue. Building the breast mound bottom up enables the surgeon to form the breast and treat the tissue dynamically. This is a powerful technique to add to the breast surgeon's surgical toolbox.

5

Breast Implant Explantation and Multi-Level Mastopexy

Out With the Old (Implant) in With Your Own (Breast)

Over the years, breast augmentation has consistently been one of the most commonly performed plastic surgery procedures. Indeed, more than 3 million breast implants have been done for primary augmentation in the United States since 2005.[53] However, recent worldwide awareness to Breast Implant Associated Anaplastic Large Cell Lymphoma (BIA-ALCL) is, understandably, leading more patients to seek plastic surgery consultation regarding the current findings and perhaps esthetically pleasing options, involving removal of the breast implants.[55] It is now clear that any surgeon, who performs esthetic or reconstructive breast surgery, will need to become increasingly familiar with techniques to manage the explantation patient.

Multiple publications have described approaches to breast auto-augmentation, designed to maximize esthetic outcomes and minimize the likelihood of complications and reoperations.[56–58] In contrast, breast implant explantation has received much less focus, leaving behind a wide and deflated breast with very little breast tissue barely resembling the former breast form.[56–58]

The Borenstein Explantation–Pexy (BEP) technique was specifically developed to recreate the breast mound bottom up, immediately after the breast implant removal, using the laterally displaced breast tissue. When applied to properly selected patients, this technique may produce an esthetically pleasing breast.

Surgical Technique

The breast is marked as in the vertical scar mastopexy procedure.

De-epithelization of an area, smaller than the pre-surgical marking, is carried out.

A peri-areolar skin incision is made, followed by electrocautery dissection down to the capsule (Fig. 5.1).

The capsule is then entered, the implant removed, and the superficial capsule is scored (Fig. 5.2).

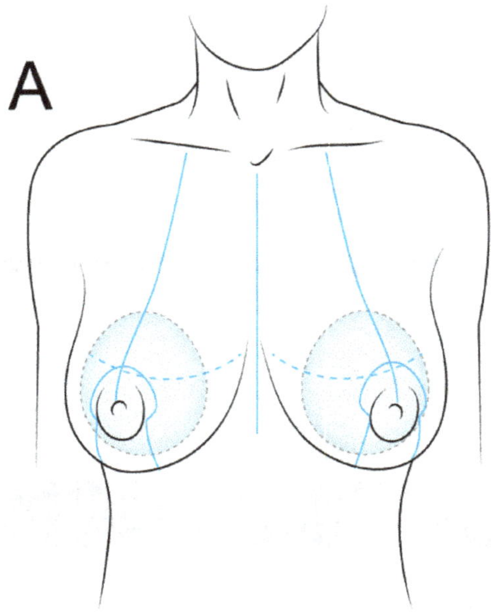

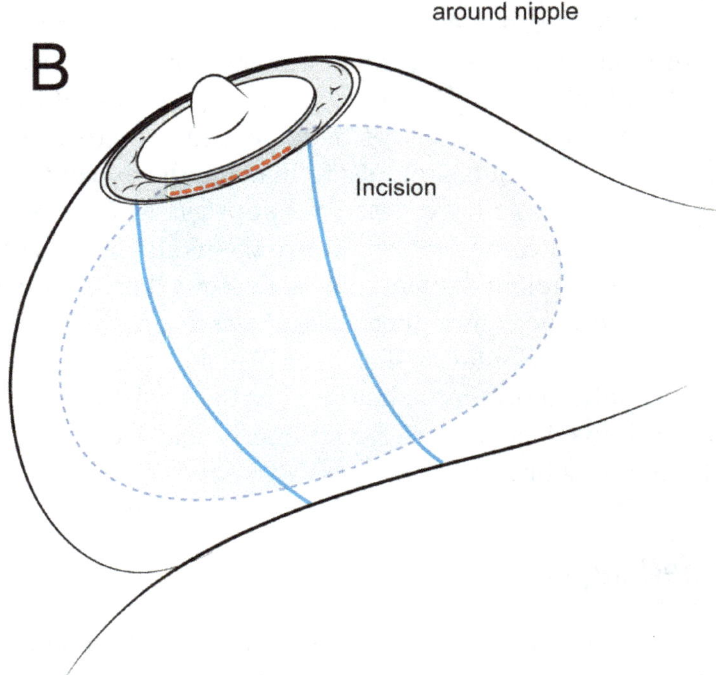

Figure 5.1. ■ Explantation pexy markings, de-epithelization, and incision. Note the peri-areolar point of access.

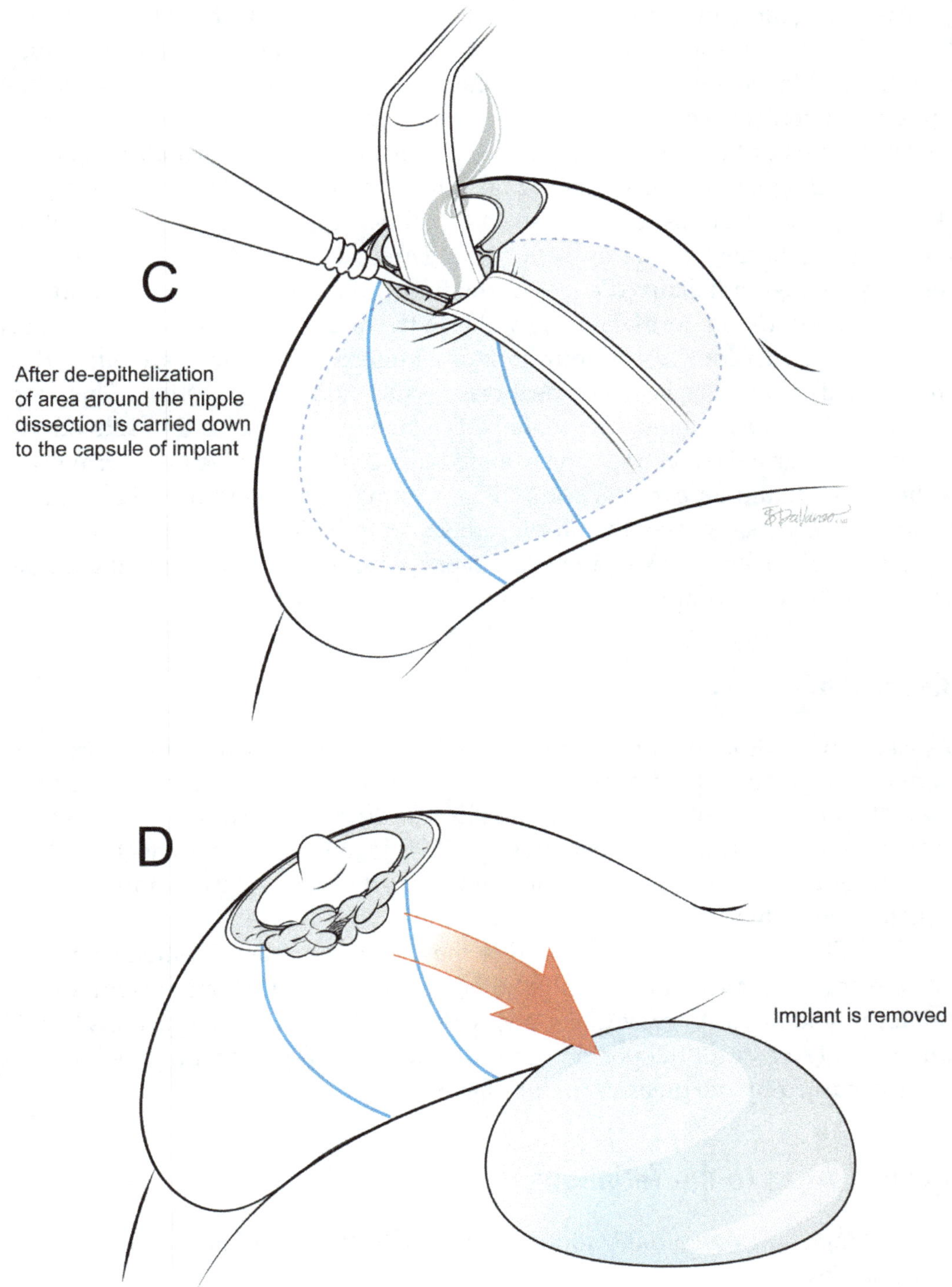

Figure 5.2. ■ **Explantation pexy removal of implant.** Note the implant space left behind.

After irrigation and careful hemostasis, 1–2 absorbable vicryl 0 (Johnson & Johnson Medical N.V., Belgium) are placed between the lateral part of the capsule and just the medial to the breast meridian, taking a good bite of the pectoralis fascia, narrowing the base of the breast and creating a pleasing lateral curve. Importantly, these sutures should not be tied down before their effect on the lateral curve of the breast is assessed. If they do not produce a pleasing curve, or if a dimple is formed, they should be placed again. Then, the opening is closed using vicryl 2-0 sutures. Depending on breast tissue thickness and quality, a central area of de-epithelization or skin and subcutaneous tissue excision is performed. Three to five inverted deep dermal sutures are put between the de-epithelialized edges of the future vertical scar. Next, the Borenstein maneuver is performed—two thin dermal flaps, similar to the facelift skin flaps, are developed on either side of the vertical incision. Two to four horizontal figures of 8 sutures are put at the freshly exposed breast tissue edges, narrowing the breast while adding projection. This step is repeated as needed. When the intended breast shape is achieved, the excess thin skin strips are cut, and the tension-free dermal edges are approximated using an absorbable intradermal suture. The patient is then seated, and an external suture is put to mark the bottom of the future areola. An inked cookie cutter is placed over the nipple–areola complex (NAC) and the surrounding skin to mark the new areola opening. De-epithelization of the rest of the areola opening is made and the insetting of the NAC is completed (Fig. 5.3).

Discussion

Breast augmentation remains the most widely performed plastic surgery procedure, with 313,735 augmentations performed during 2018 in the United States alone, a 4% rise from 2017. Removal of 29,236 breast implants was performed during 2018 in the United States, a 6% rise from 2017.[53] Growing worldwide awareness of BIA-ALCL is leading more patients to seek options involving removal of the breast implants,[55] thus substantially increasing the importance of mastering the explantation techniques.[53]

The BEP technique, described in this chapter, is suitable for patients with enough breast tissue to recreate a breast after explantation (Fig. 5.4). Patient selection is important. The ideal candidates would be the ones with supple, wide breasts. This technique aims to achieve upper pole fullness and to control the position of the NAC using horizontal obliteration of dead space formerly occupied by the breast implant (Fig. 5.4).

Tips and Tricks to the Technique

1. Markings and de-epithelization are similar to the techniques carried out in a vertical scar mastopexy.
2. Peri-areolar incision and access enable secure closure using multiple layers, control of nipple–areola position, and IMF integrity.
3. The deep absorbable sutures from the lateral capsule to the IMF just medial to the breast meridian help controlling the lateral vector of breast ptosis.

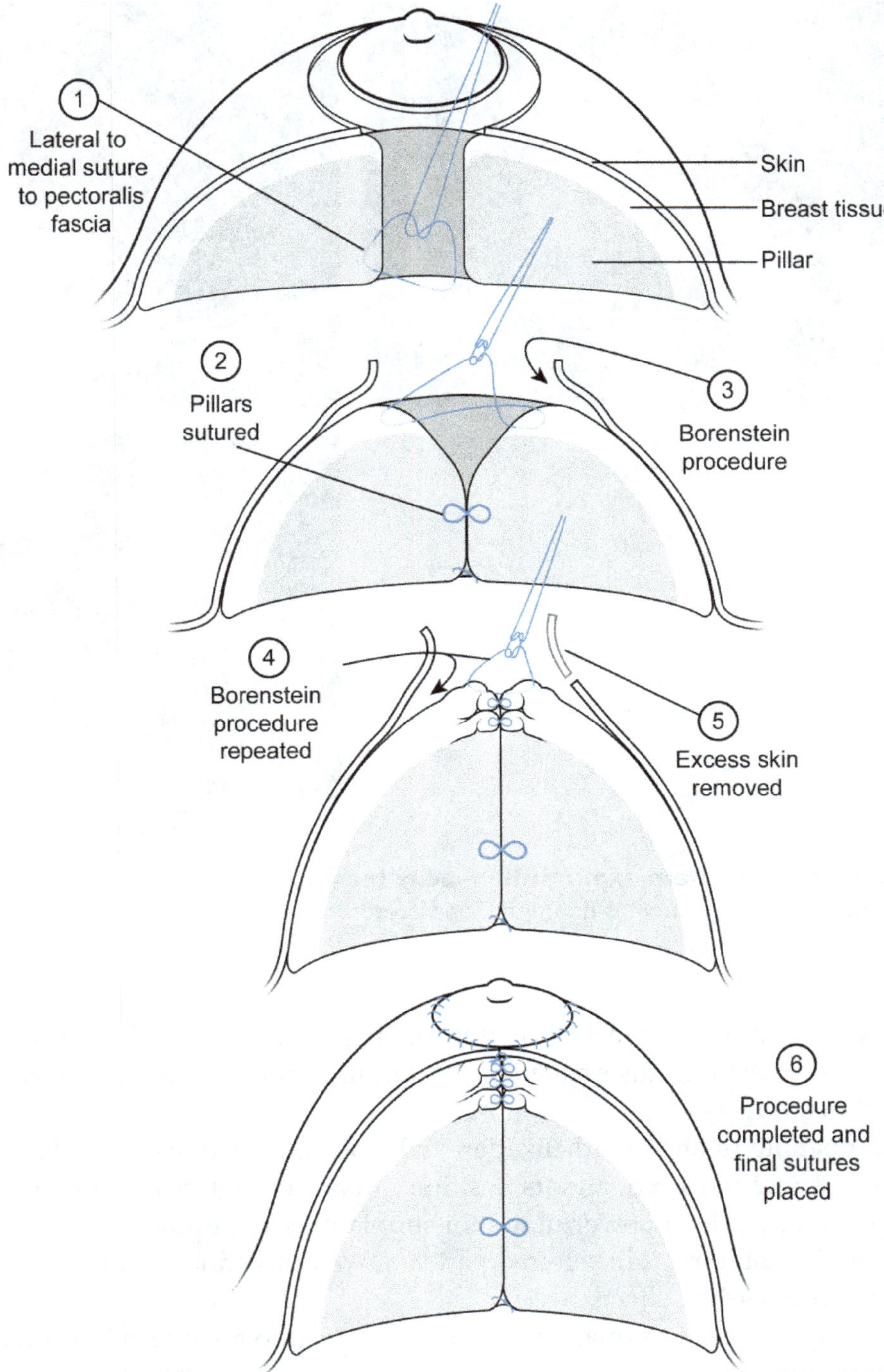

Figure 5.3. ■ Explantation pexy restructuring the breast. Note the lateral sutures to the pectoralis fascia and the progressive layered closure facilitated by the Borenstein maneuver.

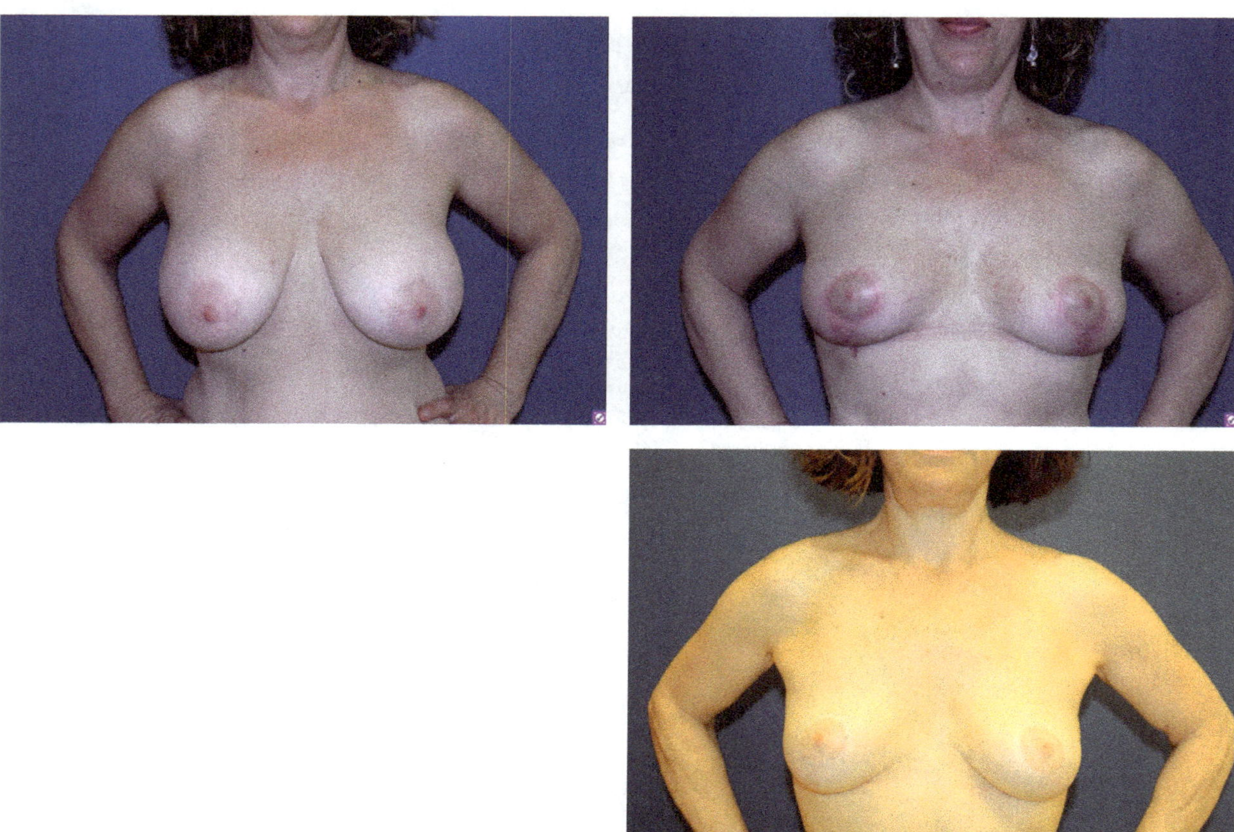

Figure 5.4. ■ Borenstein explantation–pexy technique. Before (left) and after (right) photos. Note the photos before (top left), 3 months (top right), and 6 years after (bottom right) surgery.

4. Layered closure of the invaginated breast tissue outward to the vertical scar converts breast width to projection, aids final NAC positioning, and reduces the tension of the final intradermal skin sutures.
5. NAC opening final de-epithelization and placement is done as the last step when the breast mound is reconstructed, and its position can be verified in a 3D manner.
6. Fat grafting can be a powerful tool in supplanting the upper breast pole and we would recommend combining it in selected patients. Well-placed fat of 30–50 cc can create a dramatic almost implant-like effect.
7. In our experience, fat explantation is fantastic; we do not overfill the breast and use the plane between the capsule remaining breast tissue and within the breast tissue itself.

8. Care must be taken to deposit small fat portions well-spaced as advocated by Roger Khouri and Syd Coleman.

Limitations

There are several limitations associated with the BEP technique. First, our patient selection process excludes patients with grade IV capsular contracture or patients planned for total capsulectomy. We do however suspect, based on our mastopexy and reduction experience, that the method may be applied in selected cases planned for total capsulectomy, if sufficient breast tissue remains. Second, patients with poor remaining breast tissue, radiated patients, and post-mastectomy implant-based reconstructed patients are not candidates for this procedure. In these cases, alternative methods of breast reconstruction such as local, regional, free flaps, or multiple rounds of fat transfer may be indicated.[59–61]

Conclusion

Breast augmentation remains the top plastic surgery procedure performed worldwide. Natural changes in body and breast shape, device failure, malposition, and patient preference bring more patients every year to plastic surgery explantation consultations. The BEP technique is a non-implant-based surgical option for selected patients, seeking removal of their esthetic breast implants (Figs. 5.5–5.7).

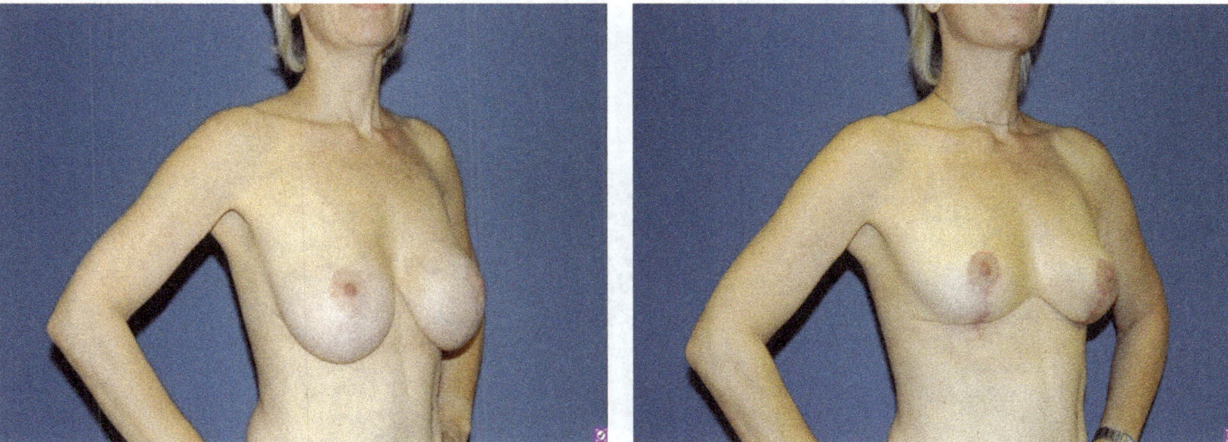

Figure 5.5. ■ Borenstein explantation–pexy technique. Before (left) and after (right) photos. Note the lateral view and created projection 6 months after surgery (right).

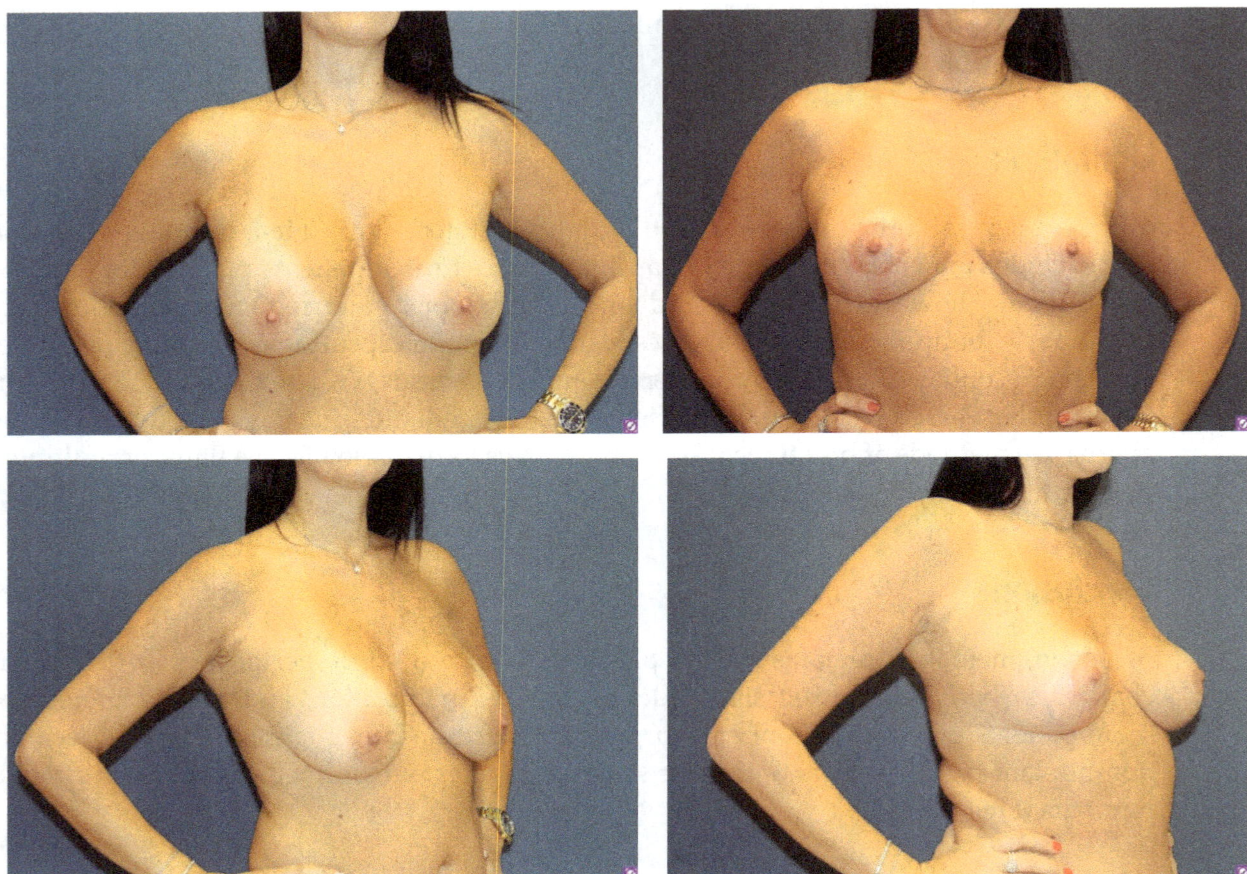

Figure 5.6. ■ **Borenstein explantation–pexy technique.** Before (left) and after (right) photos. Note asymmetry and waterfall deformity before versus the natural perky breast appearance after.

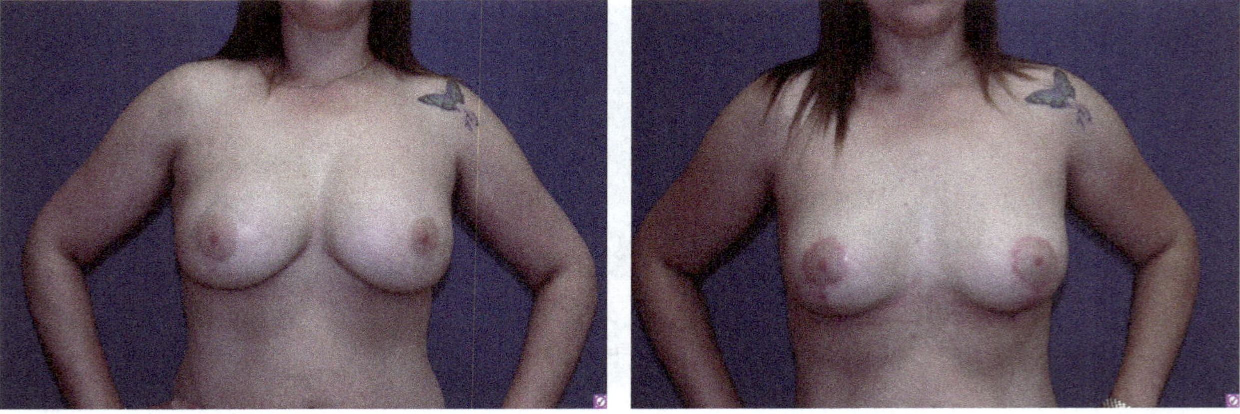

Figure 5.7. ■ **Borenstein explantation–pexy technique.** Before (left) and after (right) photos. Note a patient with beautifully augmented breast before surgery (left). Three months after explanation and mastopexy, the breasts have a natural esthetic appearance with almost augmented like projection (right). The areolas diameter was corrected on both sides as well.

6

Breast Augmentation and Multi-Level Mastopexy

First described by Gonzales-Ulloa in 1960, the breast augmentation and mastopexy procedure have fascinated many patients. The search for the ultimate stop & shop breast surgery has finally come to an end — lift and volume in a single stage, reduced cost, and less overall downtime.[62] What can go wrong? Well, a lot. Spear et al. reported that up to 23% complication rate was registered in augmentation–pexy procedures compared to 1.7% in augmentation alone,[63] pointing to an "exponential increase" in complication rates.[64] Others have labeled this procedure as a "common source of litigation."[65]

Augmentation and mastopexy work on opposing vectors. Augmentation exerts outward pressure on the skin, soft tissue envelope, and breast tissue by increasing breast volume, whereas mastopexy aims to reduce the soft tissue envelope. The goals of the two combined procedures are rarely achieved, and increased rates of complications, such as wound breakdown, nipple necrosis, flap loss, and implant exposure, are registered.[63] That said, some authors submit that a combined procedure can be performed safely and effectively.[66–71]

Here we describe an augmentation mastopexy surgical technique that aims to considerably reduce the risk for wound dehiscence and implant extrusion, using the patient's own breast tissue in a multi-layered cover over the peri-areolar implant insertion point.

Surgical Technique

Pre-operative markings are similar to those of a superior pedicle augmentation mastopexy.

De-epithelization of an area, slightly smaller than pre-surgically marked, is carried out. Next, an inferior peri-areolar skin incision is made, followed by electrocautery dissection of the subglandular pocket (Fig. 6.1).

After irrigation and careful hemostasis, the breast implant is inserted and closed using absorbable vicryl 2-0 (Johnson & Johnson Medical N.V., Belgium) (Fig. 6.2).

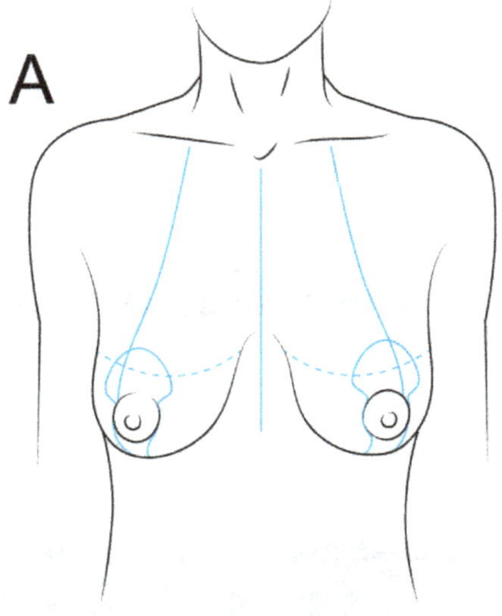

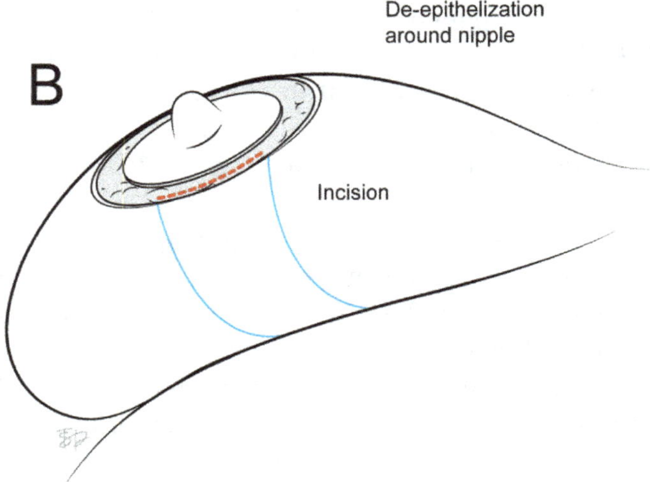

Figure 6.1. ■ Borenstein augmentation–pexy technique. (A) Surgical markings. (B) De-epithelization of an area, slightly smaller than pre-surgically marked, is carried out. Next, an inferior peri-areolar skin incision is made.

Depending on the breast tissue thickness and quality, a central area of de-epithelization or the skin and the subcutaneous tissue excision is performed. Next, the Borenstein maneuver is performed — two thin dermal flaps, similar to facelift skin flaps, are developed on either side of the vertical incision (Fig. 6.3). — Two to four horizontal figures of 8 sutures are put at the freshly exposed breast tissue edges, narrowing the breast while adding projection (Fig. 6.4).

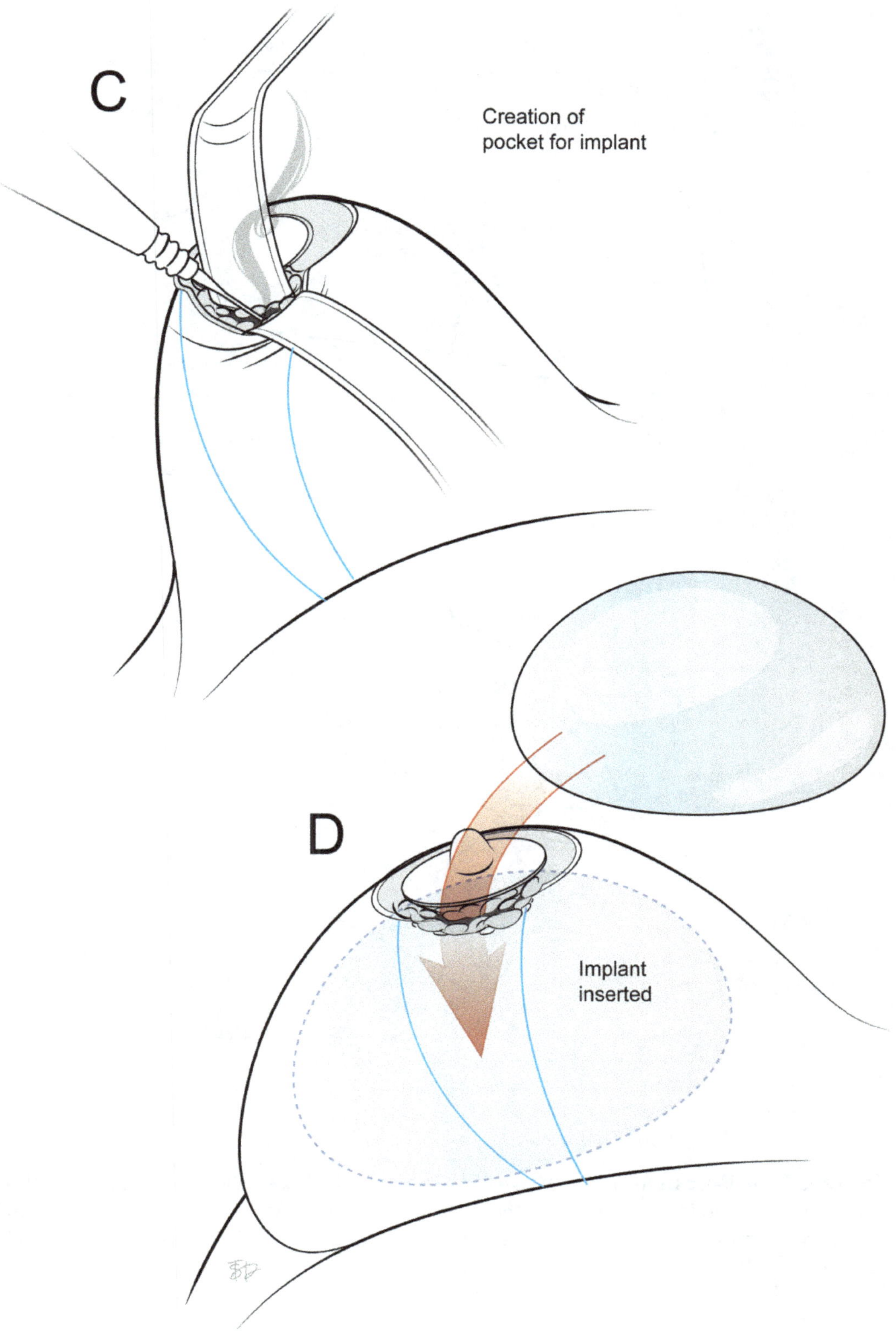

Figure 6.2. ■ **Borenstein augmentation–pexy technique.** After irrigation and careful hemostasis, the breast implant is inserted and closed using absorbable vicryl 2-0.

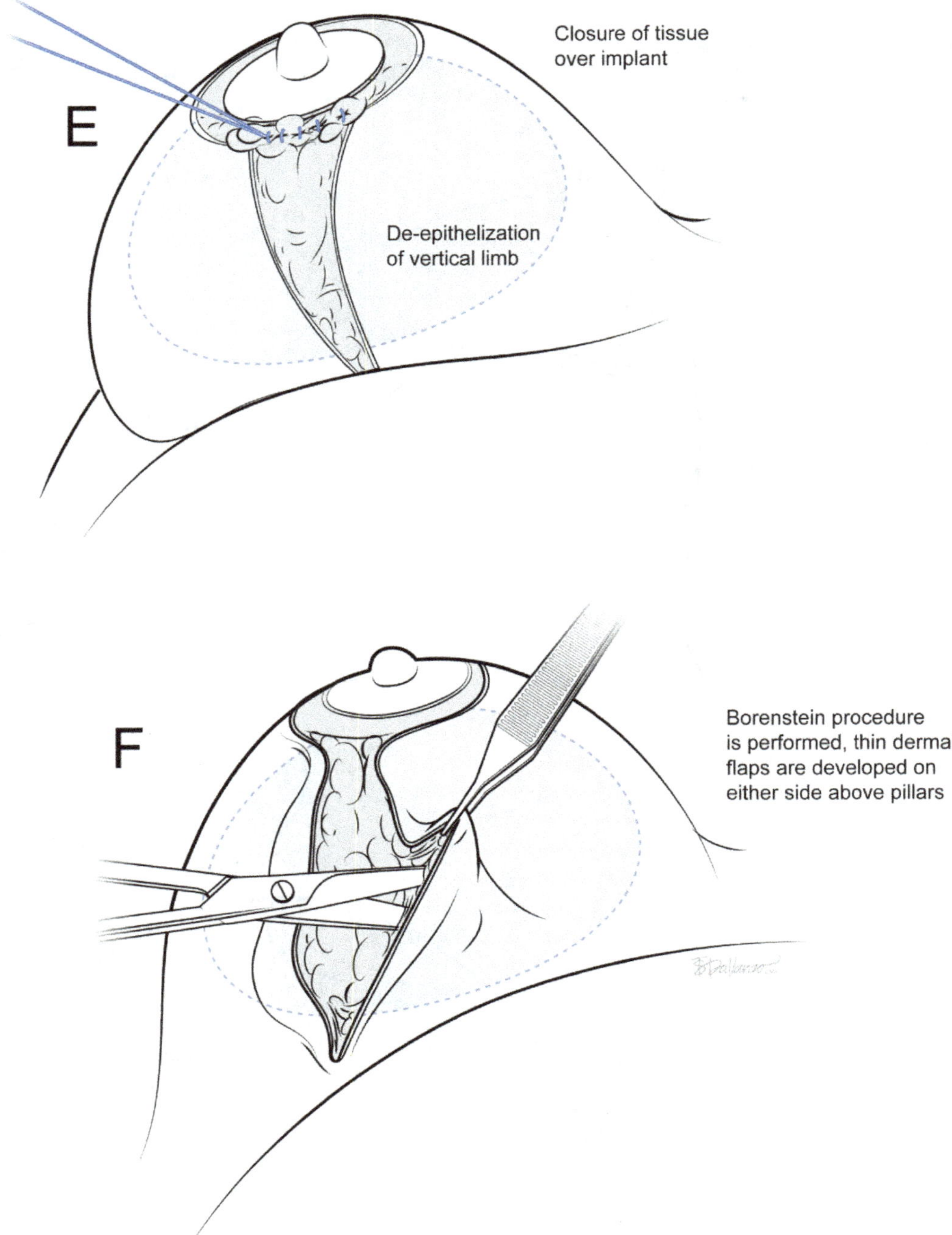

Figure 6.3. ■ Borenstein augmentation–pexy technique. The implant pocket is closed. Then, a central area of de-epithelization or the skin and the subcutaneous tissue excision is performed. Next, the Borenstein maneuver is performed — two thin dermal flaps, similar to facelift skin flaps, are developed on either side of the vertical incision.

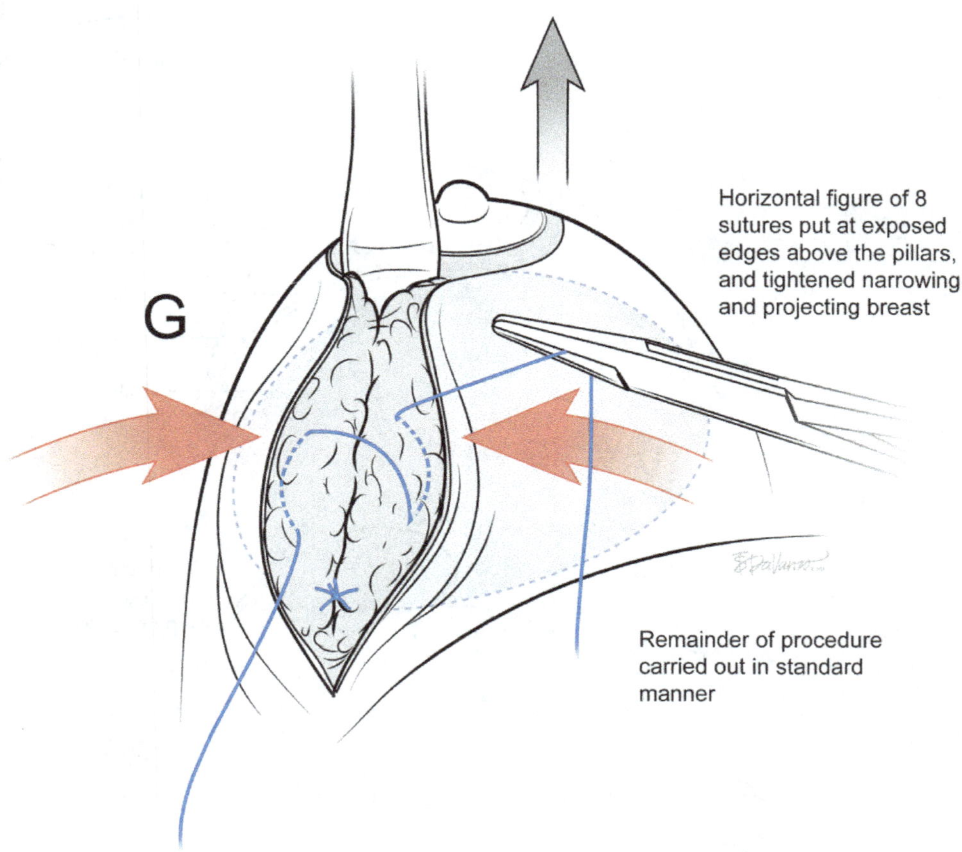

Figure 6.4. ■ Borenstein augmentation–pexy technique. Two to four horizontal figures of 8 sutures are put at the freshly exposed breast tissue edges, narrowing the breast while adding projection.

The latter step is repeated as needed. When the intended breast shape is achieved, the excess thin skin strips are cut, and the tension-free dermal edges are approximated using an absorbable intradermal suture.

The patient is then seated, and an external suture is put to mark the bottom of the future areola. An inked cookie cutter is placed over the nipple–areola complex (NAC) and the surrounding skin to mark the new areola opening. De-epithelization of the rest of the areola opening is made and the insetting of the NAC is completed (Fig. 6.5).

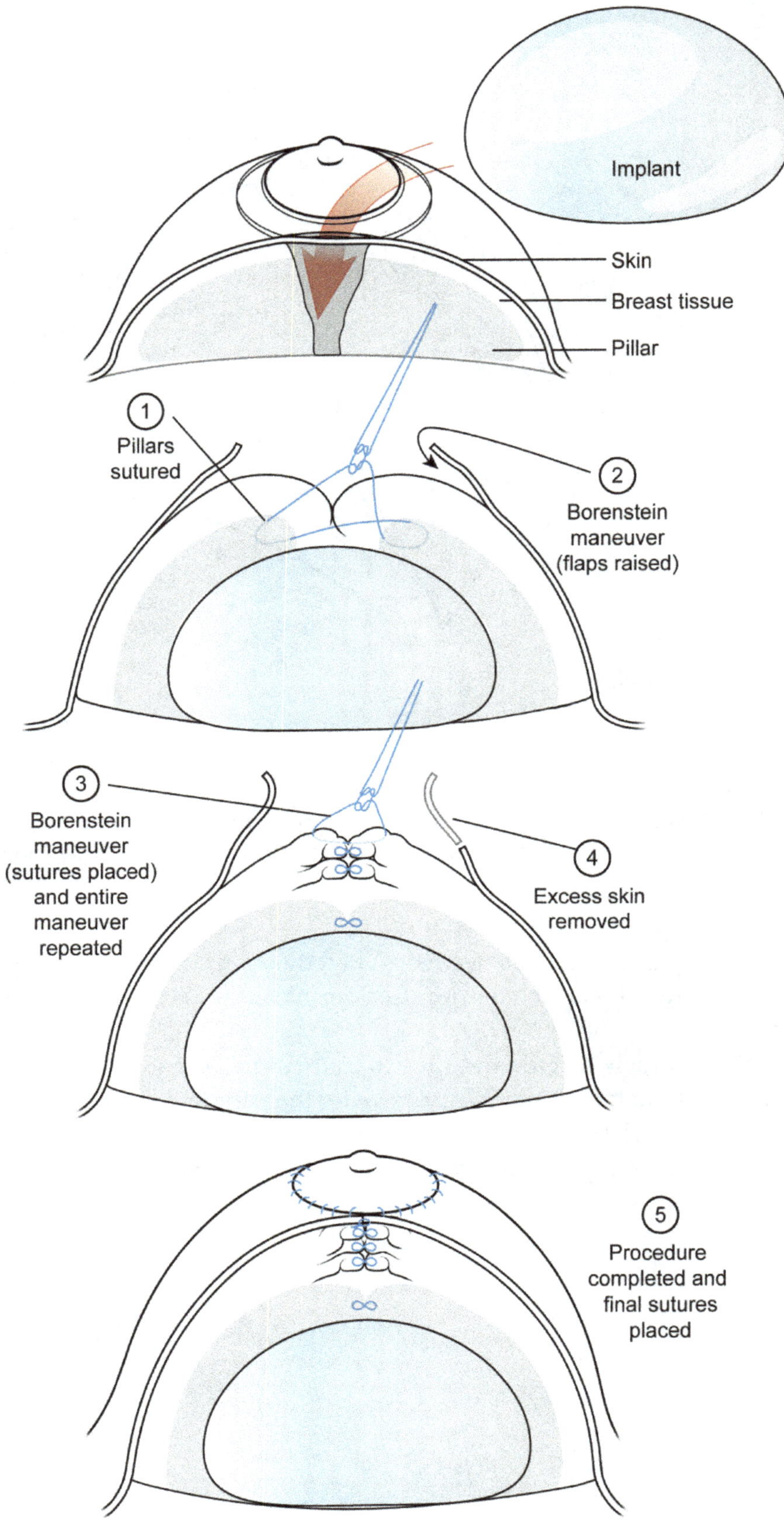

Figure 6.5. ■ Borenstein augmentation–pexy technique. Note the multi-level closure over the implant, adding protection, reinforcing the structure, and projection of the breast.

Discussion

Breast augmentation remains the most widely performed plastic surgery procedure, with 313,735 operations performed in 2018 in the United States alone, a 48% increase from 2000. Procedures of 109,638 breast lift (Pexy) were performed the same year, a 108% increase from 2000.[53]

The substantial increase in demand for both procedures underlies the appeal of combining them. Combining both procedures is an attractive option for a large number of patients but a formidable complication rate may deter the cautious surgeon.[62–65]

Over the years several authors published their experience, aimed at lowering the complication rates. In 2011, Hickman described his modification of the Goes mastopexy, using the peri-areolar approach.[67] In 2012, Gonzalez advocated his take on the circumareolar approach.[68] Other authors stressed proper technique and attention to high-tension areas in the breast after closure as key to reducing complication rates and optimizing the results.[69–71]

The Borenstein Augmentation–Pexy technique aims to considerably reduce the risk for wound dehiscence and implant extrusion by using the patient's own breast tissue in a multi-layered cover over peri-areolar implant insertion point. Additionally, upper pole fullness and control over the NAC position are achieved, applying the same maneuver of medializing the often laterally displaced ptotic breast tissue. This is accomplished by using the wide, deflated breast tissue to create projection while simultaneously adding layers of protection over the point of implant insertion (Fig. 6.6).

This technique may be applied to a wide variety of patients. However, its benefits are most evident when applied to the most challenging cases: ptotic, deflated breasts with poor skin quality. In these patients, other techniques would either fail to create projection or lead to a prohibitive complication rate, mainly wound breakdown and even implant extrusion.

The results are consistent with the senior author's (AB) breast reduction experience, where particular emphasis is given to the bottom-up restructuring of the breast mound (Fig. 6.7).

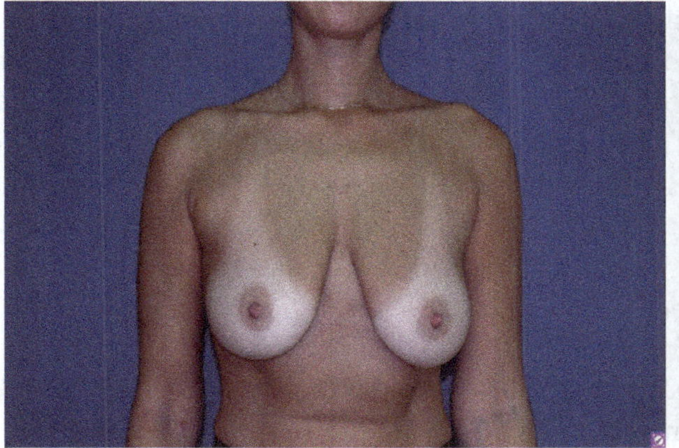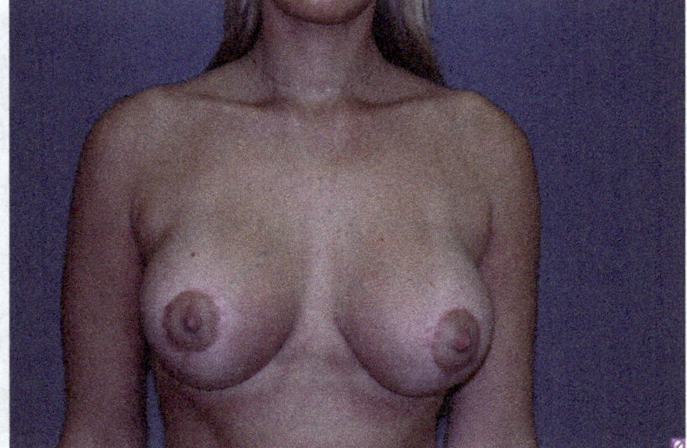

Figure 6.6. ■ **Borenstein augmentation-pexy technique.** Before (left) and 1 year after (right) surgery. Note the added fullness and fine scars.

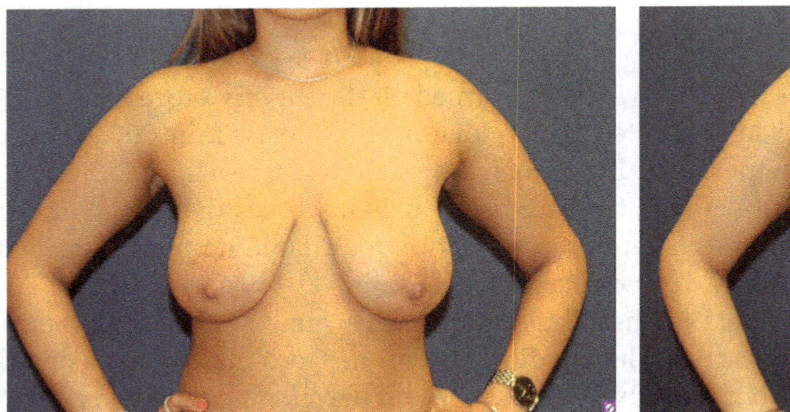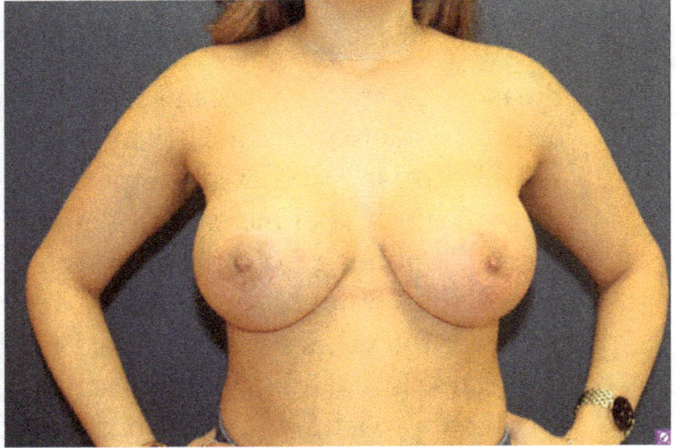

Figure 6.7. ■ **Borenstein augmentation–pexy technique.** Before (left) and 1 year after (right) surgery.

Tips and Tricks to the Technique

1. Markings and de-epithelization are similar to any superior or superior medial Pexy.
2. Peri-areolar incision and access enable secure closure using multiple tissue layers, protecting the implant and assuring the areola and IMF position integrity.
3. Medialization of the laterally displaced breast tissue implementing the lateral sutures, controlling the lateral vector of breast ptosis, and creating a pleasing new lateral slope and narrow base for the rest of the breast.
4. Layered closure of the vertical scar converts the width of the breast to projection, helps support the implants' upward displacement, adds tissue layers for protecting the implants' insertion point, aids final NAC positioning, and reduces tension from final intradermal skin sutures.
5. NAC opening final de-epithelization and placement is done as the last step when the breast mound is reconstructed, and its position can be verified in a 3D manner.
6. Fat grafting can be a powerful tool in downsizing the selected implant. Most patients are concerned regarding upper breast pole.
7. We would recommend combining it in selected patients. 30–50 cc of well-placed fat can create a dramatic almost implant-like effect. And in some cases, may enable downgrading the implant by up to 100 cc of volume.
8. In our experience fat explantation is good, but not as predictable as following explantation, perhaps due to the internal forces generated by the implant.
9. Nonetheless, we do not overfill the breast.
10. We graft the breast tissue in the upper pole from within the breast tissue flap BEFORE final areola skin closure. This enables complete control and evidence of the entering the implant pocket.
11. Care must be taken to deposit small fat portions well-spaced as advocated by Roger Khouri and Syd Coleman.

Limitations

There are several limitations associated with the Borenstein Augmentation–Pexy technique. First, this technique might not be suitable for patients with very little breast tissue, less than 1-cm pinch test. In these patients, we would consider placing the implants under the pectoralis muscle. However, if this approach is chosen, additional modification should be made to achieve homogenous soft tissue cover. Second, the peri-areolar incision may discourage some surgeons, who might consider the IMF approach for implant insertion as less likely to contaminate the implant with the lactiferous duct flora. We would caution against converting to the IMF approach while using this technique. It is our opinion that using the Borenstein maneuver for "bottom-up" breast mound reconstruction works best when the implant is inserted using the peri-areolar approach. Adding soft tissue coverage is expected to effectively reduce the risk for wound breakdown and extrusion while simultaneously reducing tension upon skin closure, which cannot be done using the IMF approach.

Conclusion

The Borenstein Augmentation–Pexy technique is a useful surgical option. It can effectively cover the implant point of insertion aiming to reduce the risk for wound breakdown. Additional benefits are medialization of the laterally displaced breast tissue to form the base of the breast, followed by converting the width of excess tissue to create a projection while simultaneously protecting the implant insertion site and progressively reducing tension from the final skin closure (Fig. 6.8).

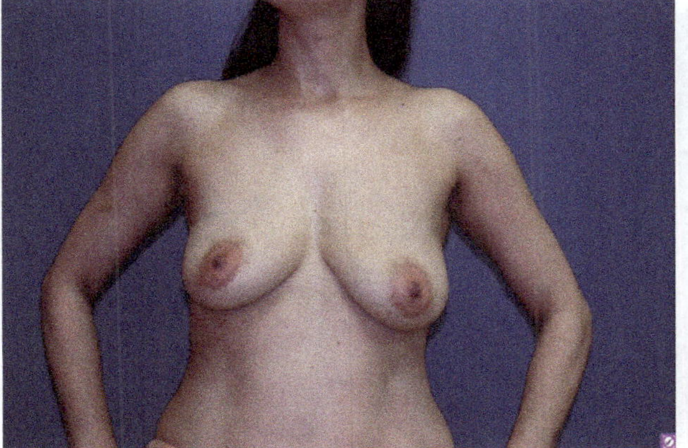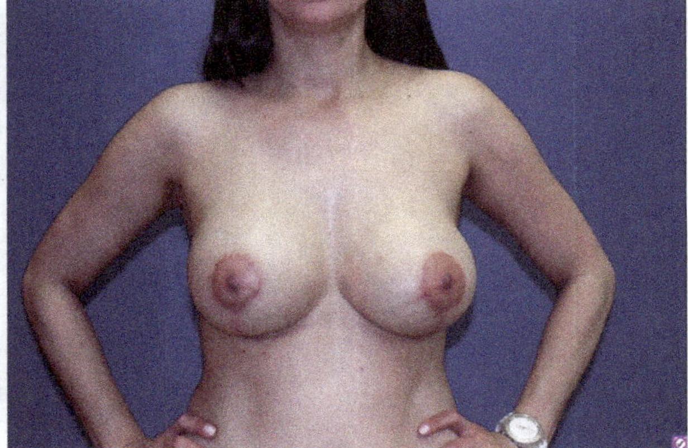

Figure 6.8. ■ Borenstein augmentation–pexy technique. Before (left) and 6 months after (right) surgery. Note asymmetrical and difficult breasts, which can be adequately filled and corrected using the technique.

7

Postoperational Breast Support

Amiram Borenstein MD, Ron Azaria MD, Roy Inbar MD and Or Friedman MD

Breast procedures are the most common procedures in plastic surgery. The 2018 ASPS statistics quote 313,735 breast augmentations, 29,236 implant removals, 109,638 breast lifts, and 43,591 breast reductions in the United States.[53] Scars are an unavoidable part of any surgery and a primary cause of concern for patients seeking esthetic breast surgery.[72] Many factors impact the post-surgical scarring. Intrinsic patient-related factors include skin quality, personal scarring tendencies, and pre-existing nutritional or medical wound healing problem.[73] Extrinsic surgeon-related factors include incision planning, atraumatic tissue handling, layered closure for tension distribution, respecting the dermal blood supply, and good epidermal opposition with minimal tension.[73] Naturally, surgeons have very little control over patient-related factors. Therefore, an open and honest discussion regarding scarring is critical in any patient evaluation and pre-surgical planning. Extrinsic factors can be managed during the surgery itself and complemented by post-surgical care.

Surgeons often use surgical tape to cover their incisions.[74] Based on the operating principles of the surgical tape, we propose a taping method that can both protect the incisions and provide better support to the breast after breast surgery.

Breast Taping Technique

Gently wipe the freshly sutured breast using damp warm lap pads, followed by dry lap pads. Several passes should be done to remove blood, serum, and fatty debris. The skin surface should not be wet or shiny at the end.

Vertical scar pattern should be taped first. Place horizontal strips of sterile porous tape (3M™, Steri-strips™) over the vertical suture line and around the nipple–areolar complex (NAC).

Thick horizontal taping should be applied second. Place the second layer of wide porous tape (3M™ Micropore™) spanning the breast. Start from the lowest part of the vertical scar, defining the inframammary fold (IMF). This step usually consists of several horizontal strips with a 50% overlap above and below the NAC.

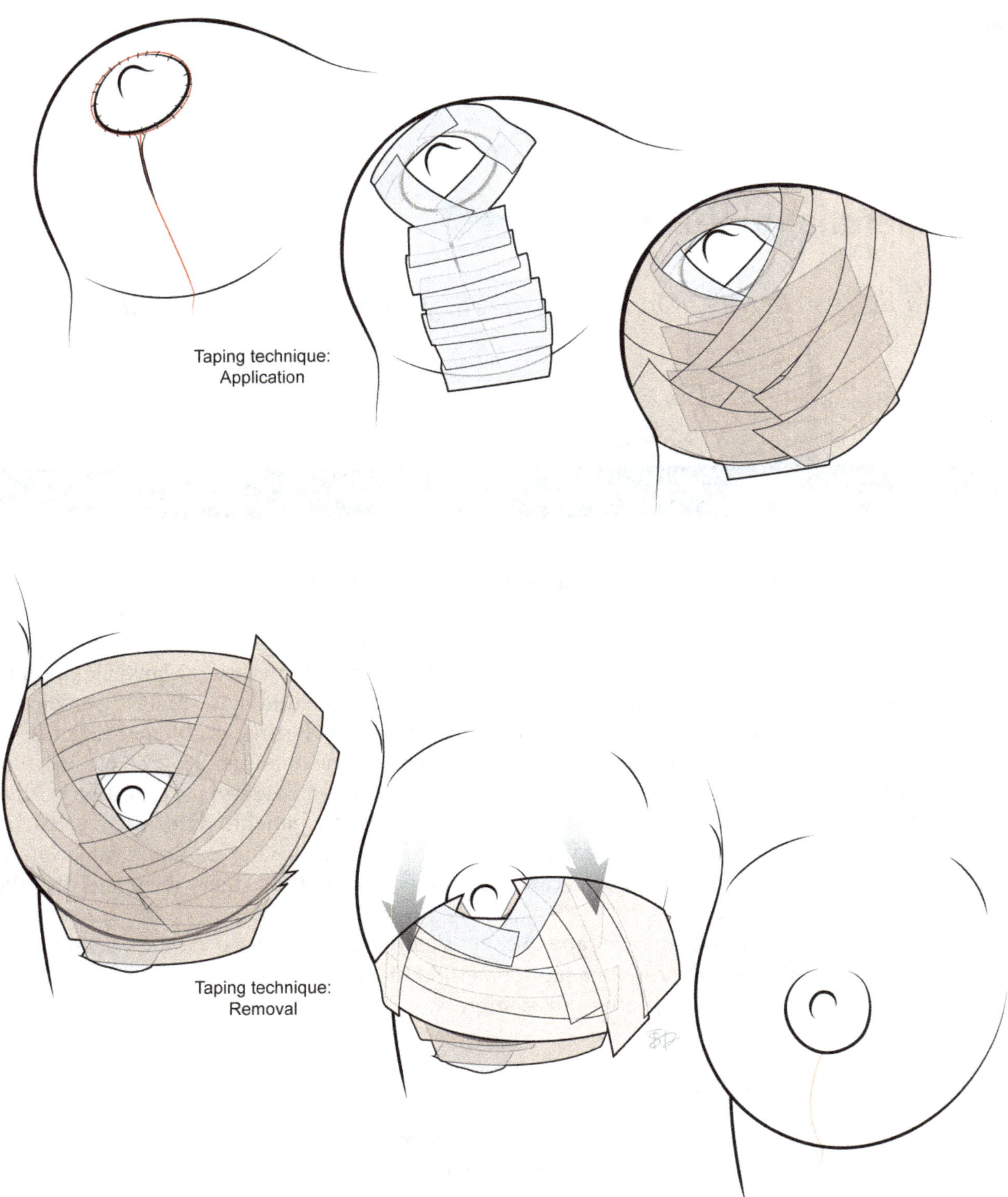

Figure 7.1. ■ Paper bra technique. Note the progressive taping adding temporary support to the reconstructed breast.

V-shaped taping should be applied third in the superomedial to the inferior-lateral direction, placing four wide porous tape strips diagonally over the breast. Then proceed in the superolateral to inferior-medial direction, placing four wide porous tape strips diagonally over the breast.

The diamond pattern is to be applied fourth to carry out medial and lateral pole taping. Here we treat the medial and lateral poles of the breast like the IMF, placing vertical strips with 50% overlap, defining the convexity of the breast and slightly suspending it by the tape (Fig. 7.1).

Follow-up

Patients are discharged with the "paper mache bra" and an unwired bra. They are seen again on POD 1, when the NAC is inspected, and the rest of the taped breast is inspected for discharge or loosening of the tape. Patients can shower with the "paper mache bra" from POD 3. The patients are inspected weekly until POD 21 when the "paper mache bra" is easily removed en-bloc with little to no discomfort to the patient (Fig 7.2).

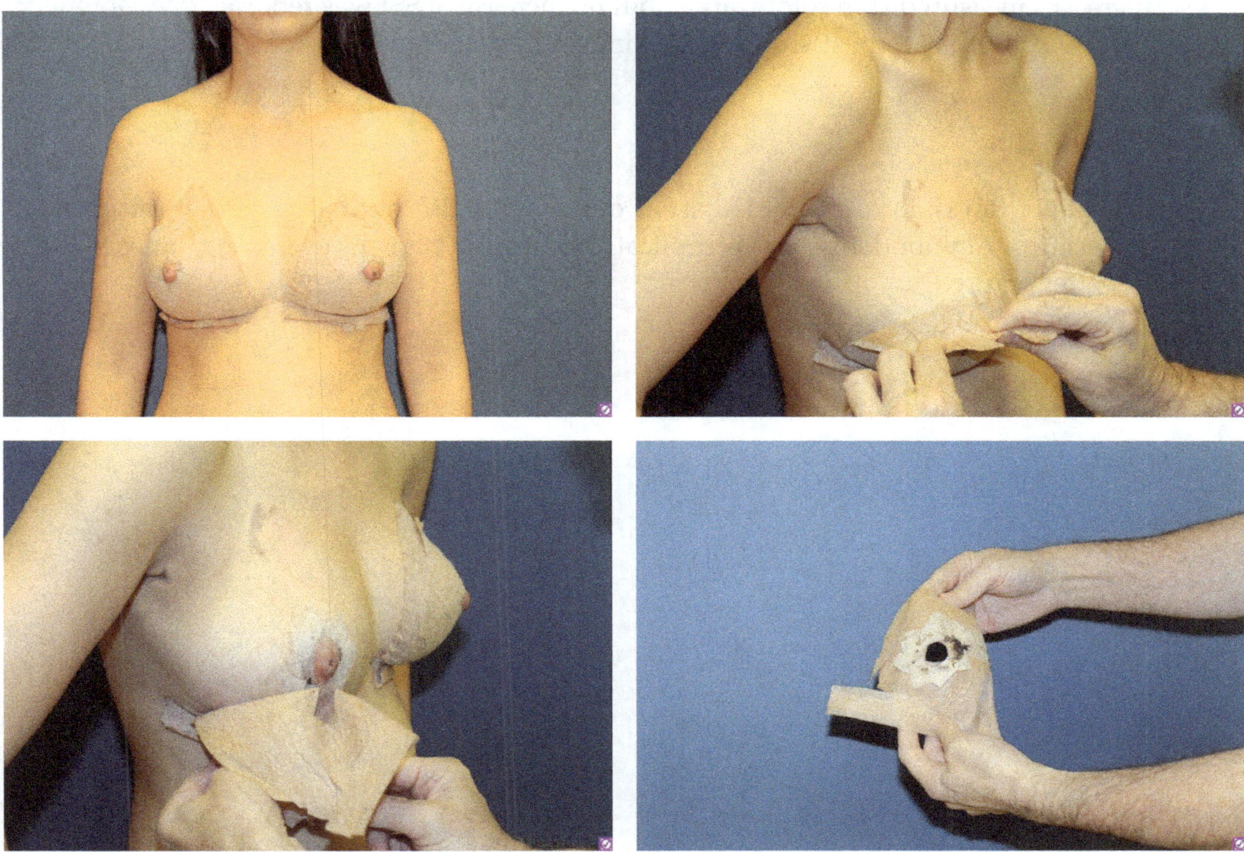

Figure 7.2. ■ Paper bra removal. Note the removal at 21 days after surgery. The paper bra is removed in one piece at the clinic.

Discussion

The breast is unique in terms of its composition and support structure. The ideal western breast is large and projected, composed mainly of soft glandular tissue and fat. The breast is supported by a series of ligaments that tether the glandular tissue and the surrounding skin envelope to the chest wall.[24,75] These ligaments are inevitably disrupted during breast surgery; therefore, the support of the breast post-op should be a vital element of any breast procedure — similar to a skin graft "tie over," or an extremity reduction and fixation.

The main advantages of the technique proposed are the custom support of the freshly reshaped breast, the ability to shower over it, and permits monitoring of the NAC.

Limitations

The limitations of this method are that it somewhat lengthens the procedure, and some might have concerns regarding skin colonization and surgical site infection (SSI). Regarding the added time, carefully cleaning and taping a single breast takes 3–5 minutes and can be done by an assistant. It has been shown by multiple level 2 and 1 studies that breast dressing up to 6 days indeed increases measured skin colonization, but no increase of SSI was reported.[76,77] Moreover, patients tend to comply with post-surgical dressing and even seem to prefer it over a daily exchange.

Conclusion

The paper bra is an inseparable part of our practice. We strongly feel that this protocol aids in lowering our minor dehiscence complication rates and perhaps even contributes to the formation of better scars.

8

Complications and Long-Term Results

The most common problem is imperfect breast shape,[50] whereas the most severe complication is necrosis.[49] Other complications include hematoma, seroma, infection, impaired healing that results in enlarged and/or displaced scars, breast asymmetry, and continued breast growth.[52] Subsequent revisions may be necessary to correct these problems; however, we would only consider revisions after at least six months have passed since the surgery.

General Considerations

Necrosis

Tension, placed on the areola, and twisting of its pedicle can change its color from a healthy shade of pink to an alarming shade of blue—the first sign of impending necrosis. Areolar necrosis is a real catastrophe in breast surgery, and all efforts should be directed toward preventing its occurrence.[45] This complication is typically noted after the areola is sutured in place, although in some rare cases it is observed during dissection. Any evidence of impending necrosis calls for immediate action in order to correct venous compression and arterial impairment. Almost all cases of necrosis are caused by impaired venous drainage and not by insufficient blood supply, at least not initially.[46]

If the areola shows signs of venous impairment at the end of the operation, the sutures should be removed, and the cause of tension or torsion will be corrected. The areola may be covered by a tepid packing for several hours and can usually be sutured back in place later. No compressive dressing is used.

We employ a stepwise approach when venous drainage restoration is required. First, the surface of the areola can be perforated with several small incisions to allow the venous blood to drain, thereby reducing the tension causing the venous impairment. Additionally, one may use topically applied heparin-soaked dressing (Heparin leech) over the incisions, up to 6 times a day, to keep the congested blood flowing. A light vaseline gauze dressing is applied to avoid crusting on the small incisions. Second, if this maneuver does not produce sufficient improvement, the sutures around the areola may be removed, permitting the areola to collapse into the breast. After 3 or 4 days, when the edema has subsided, and the natural pink color has returned, the areola can be sutured into place without further damage. Some surgeons propose to transform the areola into a free graft and relocate it to its former site, when signs of impending necrosis are spotted. However, since the dermal bed for the graft has also suffered from a venous impairment, we question whether this location would be a suitable recipient site for the graft.

If these efforts fail, it is most likely that the areolar pedicle has been damaged. The patient should be advised that a prolonged period of healing can be expected. Despite the rather alarming appearance of the breast, once the areas of glandular and fat necrosis have been excised and dressed, the wound will heal without reoperation. With the removal of necrotic tissue at each dressing change, the wound will heal by secondary intention. The surgeon should resist the temptation to return the patient to the operating room to excise tissue and re-suture the wound. If necrotic tissue has been left in place, the wound will reopen. If secondary excision is extensive, viable tissue will probably be excised, and the final size of the breast will be reduced. Patience and the application of wet or vaseline gauze dressings are the only treatment indicated. Antibiotic administration is unnecessary for a well-drained wound. The most critical and challenging task is to reassure the patient that the outcome will be much better than the initial appearances suggest.[50]

Healing, however, will not create a new areola, although some tissue may survive. With necrosis, sensitivity is forever lost, because the small nerves, innervating the areola, have been destroyed. Strangely, most patients do not mention this lack of sensation unless asked about it.[47,48,78] This is true not only after reductions with healing complications, but also after reductions that have healed uneventfully.[40] Women are much more likely to be distraught by misshapen breasts than insensitive nipples. Indeed, external appearances, i.e., shape, scars, and symmetry, are the overriding concerns.[51]

Infection hematoma and seroma

Infection does not usually occur in isolation. It frequently accompanies healing complications in a necrotic field, which is prone to bacterial growth. Early antibiotic administration is indicated.[78] Dosages are adjusted according to the results of culture studies and antibiotics can usually be discontinued after one week of treatment. Yet, establishing proper drainage, rinsing of the cavity, and debridement of the open wound are the preferred treatments.

We feel that hematomas occur mainly due to technical errors, especially following epinephrine solution infiltration, which decreases bleeding only temporarily. Hematomas are uncommon if hemostasis is ensured. However, when they do occur, we make a point of evacuating them in the operating room and ensuring a bloodless field upon closure.[46]

With appropriate dissection, seromas are no longer the problem they once were. If seromas do occur, they appear as fluctuating swellings in the lower part of the breast. Needle aspiration to remove blood-tainted fluid can be performed once or twice at one-week intervals until there is no more fluctuation. On the first aspiration, as much as 60 cc may be withdrawn. On the second time, 10–20 cc may be removed. In rare cases, a third aspiration may be indicated. This procedure is not painful, because the lower breast skin will be anesthetic for several weeks after surgery.

After aspiration, the compressive dressing is replaced, and the wound is checked in the following week. The long-term result is generally not affected, but the lower breast may remain a little more fibrous than usual for several weeks or months.

Wound dehiscence

Superficial wound dehiscence is usually caused by ischemia or infection, often in combination. If wound dehiscence follows swelling, redness, and leakage of fat or necrotic tissue, it is secondary to glandular necrosis and healing will be slower. We do not routinely operate on patients over 32 BMI, but we have noticed a trend in minor wound dehiscence in cases with extensive resections from very large breasts.[52]

Delayed Problem

Poor healing and scarring

The most severe delayed complication is poor healing that results in red and widened scars. Some crusting may form in the vertical scar. Sometimes slight widening of the scar in the lower part to the vertical suture may appear. Healing problems caused by a minor local condition such as extrusion of a subcutaneous suture can be corrected with the patient under local anesthesia several months after the initial surgical procedure.[49]

Exposure of the breasts to the sun or ultraviolet rays after surgery can make scars more noticeable because they remain pale, and for this reason, we advise patients against tanning topless.

Long-term results

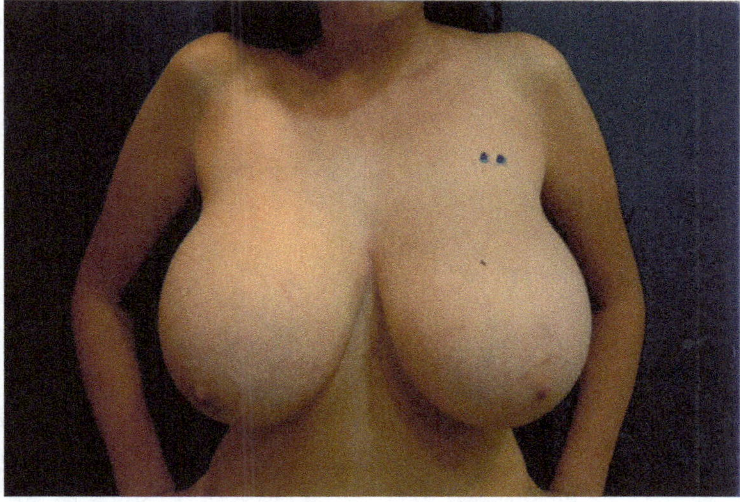

Figure 8.1. ■ Borenstein breast reduction. Before surgery.

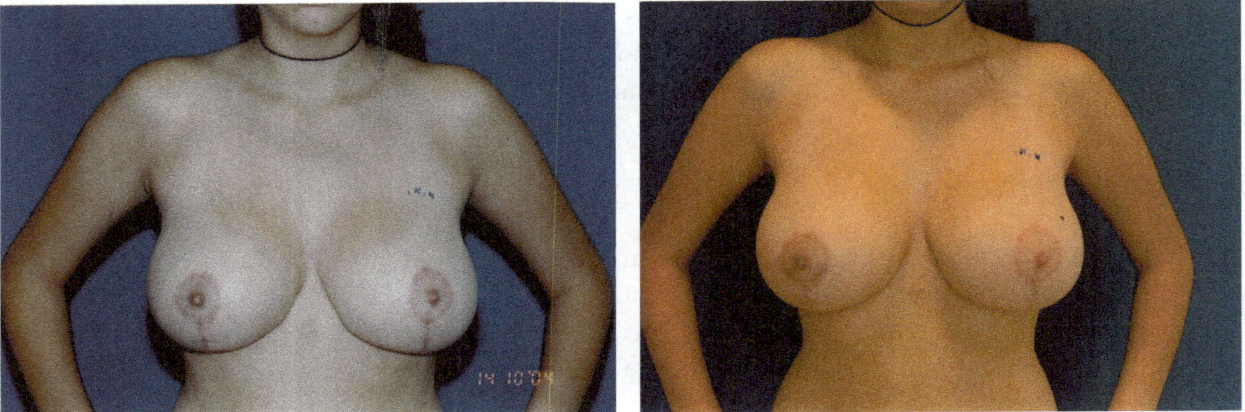

Figure 8.2. ■ **Borenstein breast reduction.** 3 months (left) and 4 years (right) after surgery.

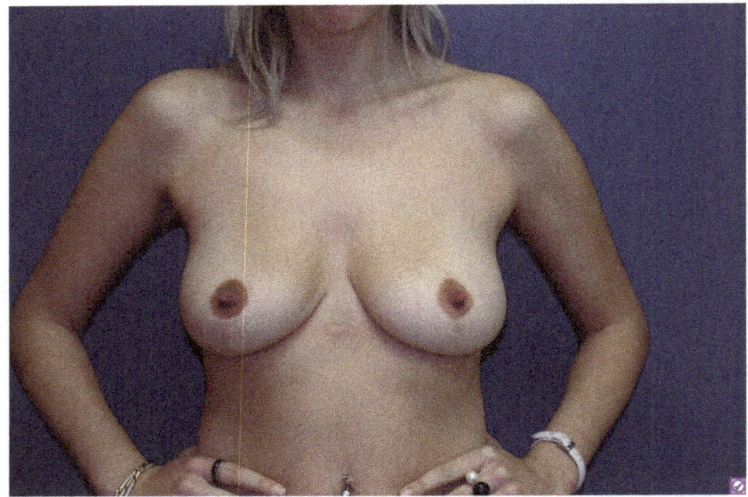

Figure 8.3. ■ **Borenstein breast reduction.** 13 years after surgery. Note that the patient had two children which she also breastfed.

9

Advanced Scar Treatments

Ofir Artzi MD and Or Friedman MD

Scars Are Like Diamonds

Ideal post-surgical scars are flat, narrow, pale, and pliable. Abnormal scars may range from hypertrophic to keloid. Post-surgical abnormal scarring with its physical sequelae (pain, itching, unattractive appearance) and resultant psychological stress can dramatically impact a patient's quality of life as well as overall patient satisfaction with medical procedures. Apart from being esthetically unpleasant, these scars are a constant reminder of the patient's past or present disease and the related surgery and can be associated with extensive functional and psychosocial morbidities.[79] Many patients seek treatment for their existing scars. In addition, the field of scar mitigation, which refers to scar treatment during the period of wound healing, aiming to minimize scarring and achieve the best esthetic outcome, has gained popularity during the past years.[80]

Scar Treatment

Numerous treatment options exist for scars including intralesional and topical medications, specialized bandages, radiation, and surgical methods. However, none has revolutionized scar treatment as much as the laser- and the energy-based technology.[80] Recognizing the various individual scar characteristics as well as patient-specific considerations (e.g. skin color) should guide the appropriate combined approach. One should be familiar with the available treatment options for the different scar components in order to maximize results.

Most scar types require several treatment sessions. During the consultation, the patient should be apprised of the possible treatment options, including the need for multiple modalities and combination therapies as well as a realistic estimate of the number of treatment sessions required. The endpoint of therapy is often determined by patient satisfaction with scar improvement.

We would like to share with you our preferred approaches for different scar types.

Mature and Stable Surgical Scars

We treat uncomplicated, stable surgical, or laceration scars with fractional lasers. These lasers split a single beam into hundreds of microbeams, creating small thermal injuries (termed microthermal zone, MTZ) while preserving the surrounding skin.[81] Normal skin remodeling proceeds from the adnexal structures as well as the intervening zones of unaltered tissue. Fractional laser devices may be either ablative or non-ablative. We prefer ablative fractional lasers on adnexal-rich skin (face) and non-ablative fractional lasers (NAFL) in adnexal-poor areas (trunk and extremities).[81–83] There are two key parameters in fractional lasers: pulse energy and density. Pulse energy correlates with the depth of penetration of the laser beam and the resultant depth of the coagulated column of tissue. Treatment density refers to the percentage of tissue that is coagulated or ablated. We mostly use fractional ablative CO_2 laser (FACL) for scar treatment. This laser is more weakly absorbed by water and vaporizes slightly thicker layers (20–30 µm) of tissue with a residual thermal damage zone of 50–130 µm.[84,85] In addition, the absorption of certain anti-scarring drugs following FACL will be highly enhanced through laser-assisted drug delivery (LADD).[86] In our experience, the energy should match the depth of the scar without exceeding scar thickness. Palpation is generally adequate to approximate scar thickness, but more precise modalities, such as ultrasound, provide a more accurate assessment of scar depth. For LADD, low-energy and low-density parameters can be used[86–88] (Fig. 9.1).

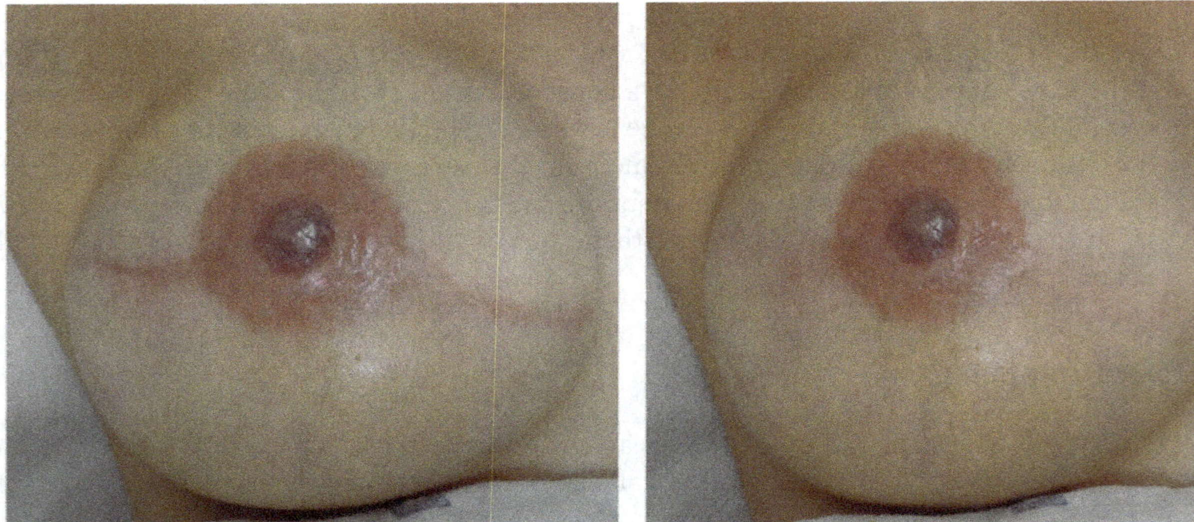

Figure 9.1. ■ Treatment of a mature stable scar. Note the reduction in height of the irregular hypertrophic scar using CO_2 laser treatment.

Erythematous and Relatively Flat Surgical Scars

A pulsed dye laser (PDL) or a potassium titanyl phosphate (KTP) laser and different intense pulse laser systems can target hemoglobin chromophore and are best utilized to alleviate the erythema associated with highly vascular post-surgical scars.[89] Also, PDL has been observed to upregulate the p53 tumor suppressor gene, inhibit cell proliferation, and reduce angiogenesis that contributes to abnormal scarring[90] (Fig. 9.2).

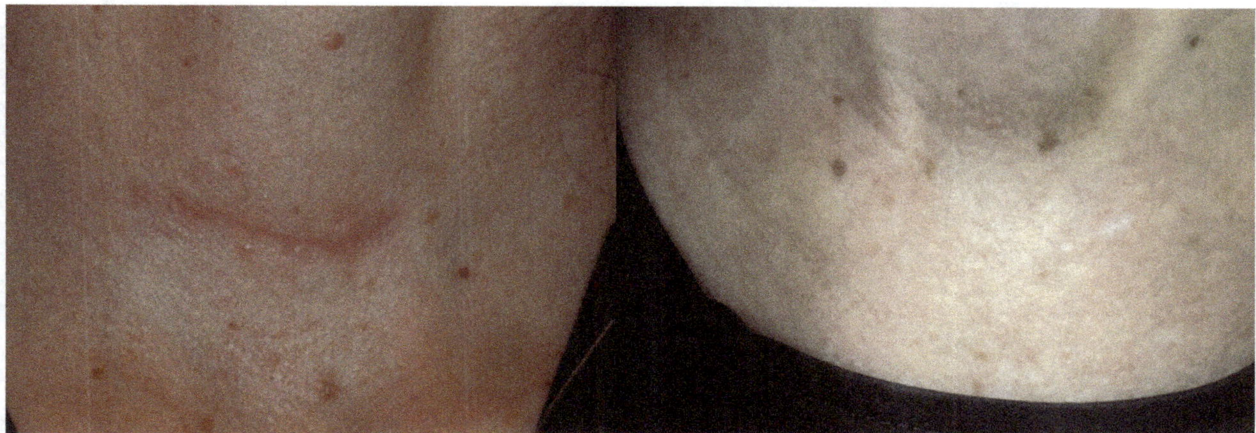

Figure 9.2. ■ Treatment of erythematous and relatively flat surgical scars. Note the marked improvement in redness that would have probably faded with time, but also the effect on the overall appearance of the final scar achieved by the modulation of the proliferation stage of scar healing. Treated using PDL.

Erythematous and Slightly Hypertrophic Post-surgical Scars

Vascular laser treatment in combination with fractional lasers is the mainstay of treatment for such scars.[91–93] NAFL is preferred and will provide a good outcome. Between treatments, occlusive, high-pressure dressings are recommended (Fig. 9.3).

Mature/Stable (Non-Erythematous) Hypertrophic Scars

FACL treatment effectively improves hypertrophy in stable scars of any thickness.[84,85] FACL also enhances topical drug delivery, as ablated channels permit enhanced penetration into deeper layers of the dermis.[91] We highly recommend the immediate CO_2 laser application of topical corticosteroids and/or 5-FU products to improve the texture, hypertrophy, contractures, and dyschromia.[87,88] A novel non-laser drug delivery system, Tixel (NOVOXEL ltd, Israel), can be used for relatively thin, hypertrophic scars or in children.[94,95] This technology combines thermal energy with motion. The system consists of a titanium tip, heated to 400°C. The tip is advanced to contact the skin. Therefore, the ablative effect on the skin is that of physical contact and transduction of heat to the superficial layers of the skin, as opposed to the laser energy that targets chromophores within the skin and heats them. Immediately after skin treatment, triamcinolone acetonide (40 mg/mL) and 5-fluorouracil (50 mg/mL) mixed at a 1:9 ratio are topically applied to the treatment area at a dose of 1 cc/cm² with occlusion.

Atrophic Scars

Atrophic scar treatment is focused on inducing neocollagenesis to reduce scar depth and improve skin texture. We find that ablative fractional resurfacing (AFR) effectively improves skin texture and surface irregularity in post-burn and post-traumatic atrophic scars and is beneficial compared to NAFL or radiofrequency-based treatment.[96] Low-energy, low-density AFR followed

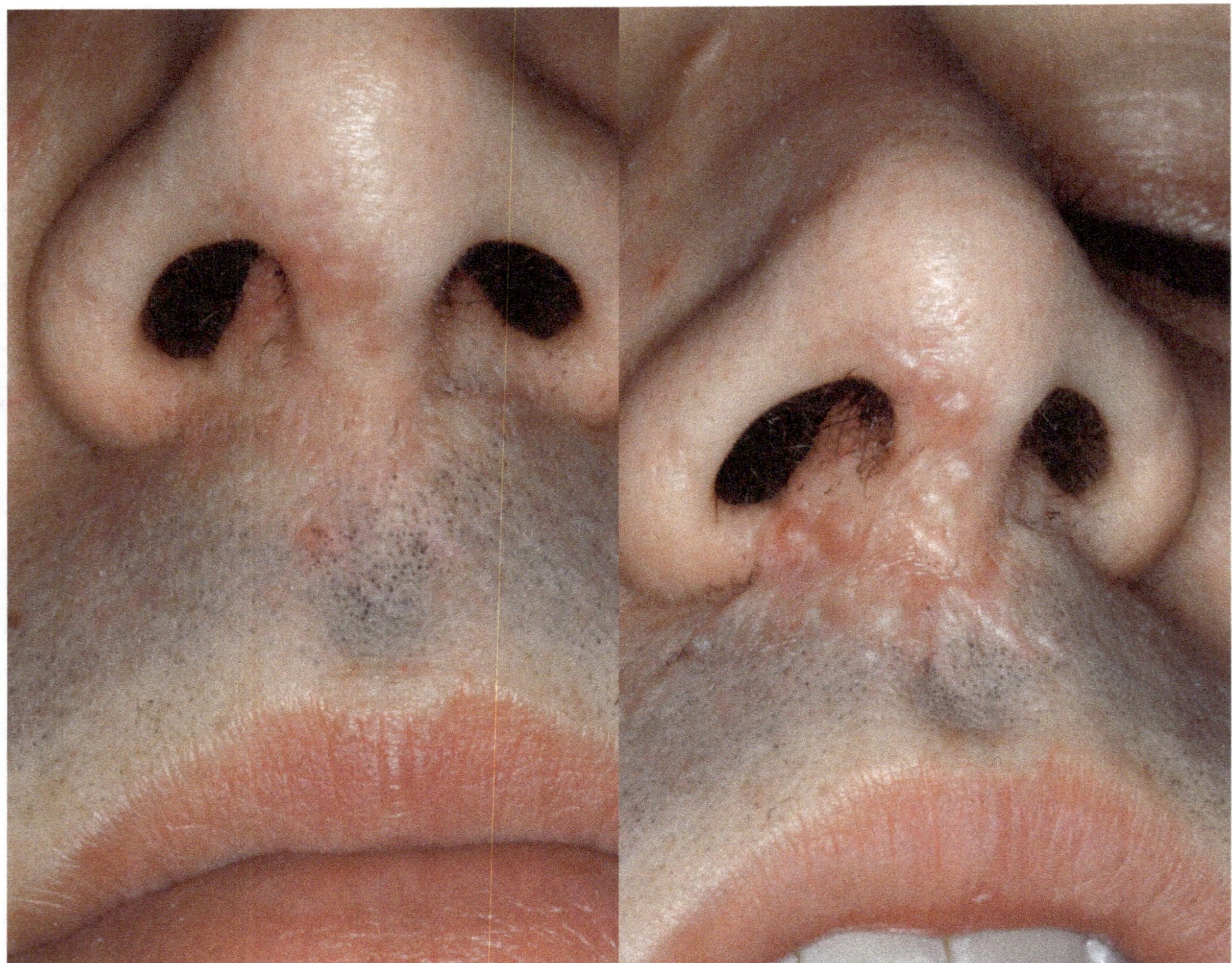

Figure 9.3. ■ Treatment of erythematous and hypertrophic surgical scars. Note the improvement in redness and reduction in height achieved by a combined PDL, CO_2, and silicone sheeting.

by the application of topical poly-l-lactic acid (PLLA) (Sculptra; Valeant Esthetics, Quebec, Canada) have been observed to stimulate collagen production by fibroblasts[97] (Fig. 9.4).

Hyperpigmented Scars

Hyperpigmented scars result from the deposition of either melanin (more common) or hemosiderin. Our experience with the picosecond laser for the treatment of hyperpigmented scarring is promising, exhibiting satisfactory results (Fig. 4.4) with a low side effect and pain profile and minimal downtime. We recommend the use of NAFL,[98] mainly the fractional 1064-nm handpiece with moderate-level fluences.[99] The patient should also be instructed to apply anti-bleaching agents twice daily as well as sunscreen for a few months (Fig. 9.5).

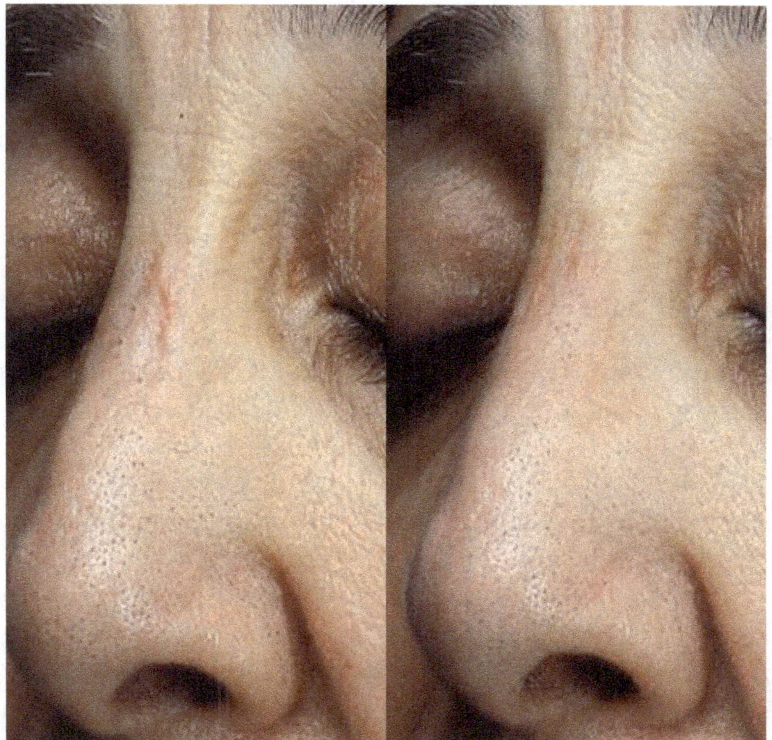

Figure 9.4. ■ **Treatment of atrophic surgical scars.** Note the improvement in contour and blurring of the sharp scar edges achieved by combined injectable poly-l-lactic acid (PLLA) and ablative fractional resurfacing (AFR).

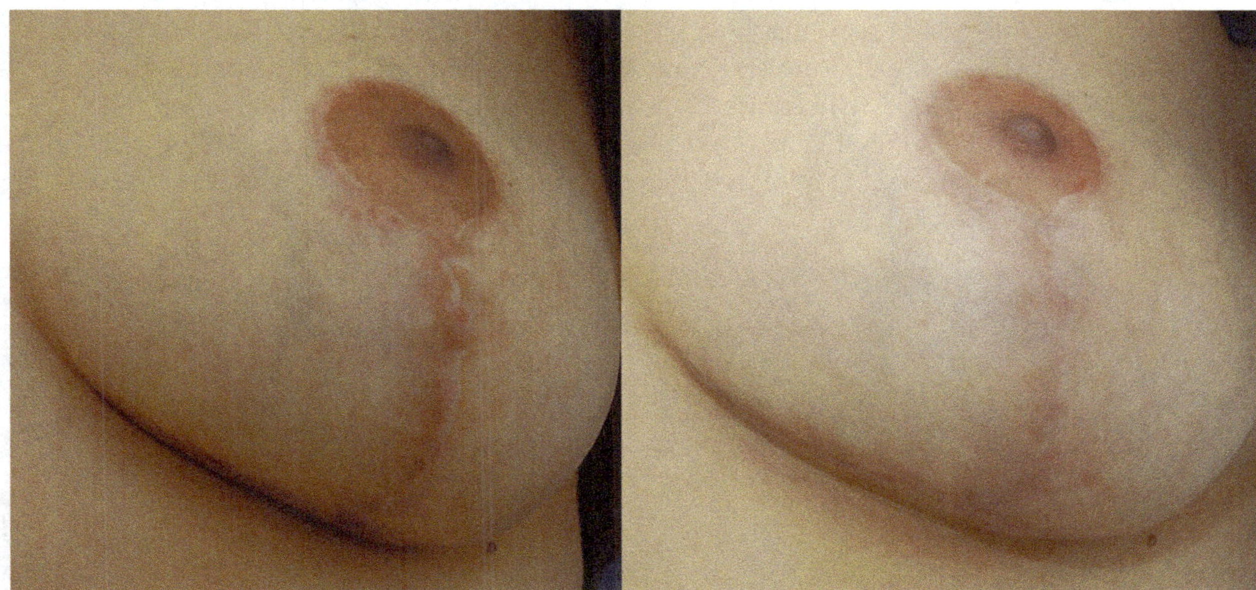

Figure 9.5. ■ **Treatment of hyperpigmented surgical scars.** Note the improvement in color using a Picosecond laser.

Hypopigmented Scars

Both AFR and NAFR improve the color and texture of hypopigmented scars. Adding a topical prostaglandin analog can further enhance the repigmentation of hypopigmented scars.[100,101] The injection of different cell suspensions coupled with Narrowband Ultraviolet B (NBUVB) phototherapy might be beneficial as well.[102]

Immature Scar or Scar Mitigation

Treatment of surgical wound before scar formation is considered preventive and is now gaining popularity. As we mentioned in Chapter 7, we consider breast taping an inseparable part of breast surgery. Since we have started breast taping, we have seen a dramatic reduction in wound breakdowns. Also, it is our opinion that the taping helps further reduce the tension on the scars in the critical time of its formation. Additional efforts to minimize scarring should be employed in high-risk patients. As for timing, most studies indicate that early, pre-scar laser treatment close to suture removal (2–4 weeks post-surgery) had the most optimal final cosmetic result.[103–106] Recent publications demonstrated the advantage of using both vascular and FACL lasers in a successive manner to achieve a better outcome. PDL or KTP is best used to treat the highly vascular post-surgical scars.[107] Also, in addition, PDL has been observed to upregulate p53 tumor suppressor gene, inhibit cell proliferation, and reduce angiogenesis that contributes to abnormal scarring.

For patients interested in further scar minimization, we offer our published protocol that was proven initially on lumpectomy scars. For taped breast, we suggest starting the treatment on POD 21 when the tape is removed from the breasts. The treatment consists of PDL immediately followed by focal FACL once monthly for three consecutive months.[107] The actual treatment time is 10 minutes. We use the following parameters: 595-nm PDL (Perfecta, Syneron-Candela, Wayland, MA) using a 7-mm spot size, 0.45-ms pulse duration, and energy fluence of 4–6 mJ/cm^2; 10,600-nm FACL (Ultrapulse Encore, Lumenis Ltd., Yokne'am, Israel) at the following settings: fluence 12.5–17.5 mJ and 5% density. The FACL treatment is performed only on the edges of the wound, on areas of observed skin tension, and on elevated or uneven surfaces (Fig. 9.6).

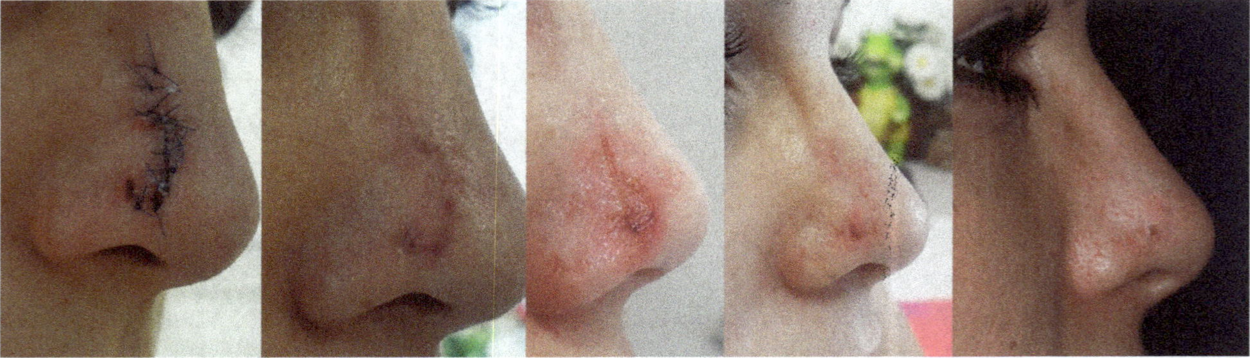

Figure 9.6. ■ Treatment of an immature surgical scar. Note the dramatic effect of planned scar mitigation using combined CO_2 and PDL laser treatments starting from suture removal.

Conclusion

As with the paper bra (Chapter 7), scar management and mitigation are an inseparable part of our practice. Great advances have been made in recent years that make scar management easier and more accessible than ever. Like diamonds, scars are forever. We feel that managing them should be a priority for any practicing surgeon.

References

1. Mundy LR, Homa K, Klassen AF, Pusic AL, Kerrigan CL. (2017) Understanding the health burden of macromastia: normative data for the BREAST-Q reduction module. *Plast Reconstr Surg.* **139**(4):846e–853e. doi:10.1097/PRS.0000000000003171

2. Wise RJ. (1956) A preliminary report on a method of planning the mammaplasty. *Plast Reconstr Surg (1946).* **17**(5):367–375. doi:10.1097/00006534-195605000-00004

3. Lejour M. (1994) Vertical mammaplasty and liposuction of the breast. *Plast Reconstr Surg.* **94**(1):100–114. doi:10.1097/00006534-199407000-00010

4. Pitanguy I. (1967) Surgical treatment of breast hypertrophy. *Br J Plast Surg.* **20**(1):78–85. doi:10.1016/s0007-1226(67)80009-2

5. Lassus C. (1970) A technique for breast reduction. *Int Surg.* **53**(1):69–72.

6. Hammond DC. (1999) Short-scar periareolar-inferior pedicle reduction (spair) mammaplasty. *Oper Tech Plast Reconstr Surg.* **6**(2):106–118. doi:10.1016/S1071-0949(99)80038-9

7. Asplund OA, Davies DM. (1996) Vertical scar breast reduction with medial flap or glandular transposition of the nipple-areola. *Br J Plast Surg.* **49**(8):507–514. doi:10.1016/S0007-1226(96)90126-5

8. Hall-Findlay EJ. (1999) A simplified vertical reduction mammaplasty: shortening the learning curve. *Plast Reconstr Surg.* **104**(3):748–759; discussion 760–3. doi:10.1097/00006534-199909030-00020

9. Lejour M, Abboud M. (1990) Vertical mammaplasty without inframammary scar and with breast liposuction. *Semin Plast Surg.* **4**(02):67–90. doi:10.1055/s-2008-1080455

10. Elbaz J. (1975) Technique de plastie mammaire par cicatrice En J. *Ann Chir Plast.* **20**(2):101–111.

11. Bozola A, Oliveira M, Sanches V, Miura O, D'Andrea S. (1982) Mamoplastia em L: contribuicao pessoal. *Revista da AMRIGS.* **26**(3):207–214.

12. Meyer R, Kesselring UK. (1979) Various dermal flaps with L-shaped suture line in reduction mammaplasty. *Aesthetic Plast Surg.* **3**(1):41–46. doi:10.1007/BF01577835

13. Chiari AJ. (1992) The L short-scar mammaplasty: a new approach. *Plast Reconstr Surg.* **90**(2):233–246. doi:10.1097/00006534-199290020-00011

14. Lassus C. (1981) New refinements in vertical mammaplasty. *Chir Plastica.* **6**(2):81–86. doi:10.1007/BF00289632

15. Marchac D, Sagher U. (1988) Mammaplasty with a short horizontal scar. Evaluation and results after 9 years. *Clin Plast Surg.* **15**(4):627–639.

16. Dartigues L. (1925) Le traitement chirurgical du prolapsus mammaire. *Arch Franco-Belge Chir.* **28**:313.

17. Arie G. (1957) Una nueva tecnica de mastoplastia. *Rev Latinoam Cir Plast.* **3**(1):23–31.

18. Converse J. (1977) *Reconstructive Plastic Surgery: Principles and Procedures in Correction, Reconstruction and Transplantation.* 2nd ed. Philadelphia, PA, WB Saunders.

19. Lassus C. (1987) Breast reduction: evolution of a technique — a single vertical scar. *Aesthetic Plast Surg.* **11**(2):107–112. doi:10.1007/bf01575495

20. Ramsay D, Kent J, Hartmann R, Hartman P. (2005) Anatomy of the lactating human breast redefined with ultrasound imaging. *J Anat.* **206**(6):525–534. doi:10.1111/j.1469-7580.2005.00417.x

21. Cooper A. (1840) *On the Anatomy of the Breast, by Sir Astley Paston Cooper, 1840.* Rare Medical Books. Thomas Jefferson University. https://jdc.jefferson.edu/cooper/. Accessed December 2, 2019.

22. Stuzin JM, Baker TJ, Gordon HL. (1992) The relationship of the superficial and deep facial fascias: relevance to rhytidectomy and aging. *Plast Reconstr Surg.* **89**(3):441–449; discussion 450–451. doi:10.1097/00006534-199203000-00008

23. Bayati S, Seckel BR. (1995) Inframammary crease ligament. *Plast Reconstr Surg.* **95**(3):501–508. doi:10.1097/00006534-199503000-00010

24. Rehnke RD, Groening RM, Van Buskirk ER, Clarke JM. (2018) Anatomy of the superficial fascia system of the breast: a comprehensive theory of breast fascial anatomy. *Plast Reconstr Surg.* **142**(5):1135–1144. doi:10.1097/PRS.0000000000004948

25. Brinkman RJ, Hage JJ. (2016) Andreas Vesalius' 500th anniversary: first description of the mammary suspensory ligaments. *World J Surg.* **40**(9):2144–2148. doi:10.1007/s00268-016-3481-6

26. Haagenson C. (1971) Anatomy of the mammary gland, in *Diseases of the Breast.* 2nd ed. Philadelphia, PA, Saunders; 16–17.

27. Vesalius A. (2007) *On the Fabric of the Human Body by Andreas Vesalius. Book V: The Organs of Nutrition and Generation.* Novato, CA, Norman Publishing. http://www.historyofscience.com/norman-publishing/anatomy/vesalius.php. Accessed December 2, 2019.

28. Cunningham L. (1977) The anatomy of the arteries and veins of the breast. *J Surg Oncol.* **9**(1):71–85. doi:10.1002/jso.2930090112

29. Würinger E, Mader N, Posch E, Holle J. (1998) Nerve and vessel supplying ligamentous suspension of the mammary gland. *Plast Reconstr Surg.* **101**(6):1486–1493. doi:10.1097/00006534-199805000-00009

30. Farina MA, Newby BG, Alani HM. (1980) Innervation of the nipple-areola complex. *Plast Reconstr Surg.* **66**(4):497–501. doi:10.1097/00006534-198010000-00001

31. Matousek SA, Corlett RJ, Ashton MW. (2014) Understanding the fascial supporting network of the breast: key ligamentous structures in breast augmentation and a proposed system of nomenclature. *Plast Reconstr Surg.* **133**(2):273–281. doi:10.1097/01.prs.0000436798.20047.dc

32. Davison SP, Mesbahi AN, Ducic I, Sarcia M, Dayan J, Spear SL. (2007) The versatility of the superomedial pedicle with various skin reduction patterns. *Plast Reconstr Surg.* **120**(6):1466. doi:10.1097/01.prs.0000282033.58509.76

33. Cardenas-Camarena L, Vergara RJ. (2001) Reduction mammaplasty with superior-lateral dermoglandular pedicle: another alternative. *Plast Reconstr Surg.* **107**(3):693–699. doi:10.1097/00006534-200103000-00007

34. Mallucci P, Branford OA. (2015) Shapes, proportions, and variations in breast aesthetic ideals: the definition of breast beauty, analysis, and surgical practice. *Clin Plast Surg.* **42**(4):451–464. doi:10.1016/j.cps.2015.06.012

35. Temple CL, Hurst LN. (1999) Reduction mammaplasty improves breast sensibility. *Plast Reconstr Surg.* **104**(1):72–76. doi:10.1097/00006534-199907000-00009

36. Hamdi M, Greuse M, DeMey A, Webster MHC. (2001) A prospective quantitative comparison of breast sensation after superior and inferior pedicle mammaplasty. *Br J Plast Surg.* **54**(1):39–42. doi:10.1054/bjps.2000.3456

37. Mofid MM, Dellon LA, Elias JJ, Nahabedian MY. (2002) Quantitation of breast sensibility following reduction mammaplasty: a comparison of inferior and medial pedicle techniques. *Plast Reconstr Surg.* **109**(7):2283–2288. doi:10.1097/00006534-200206000-00018

38. Godwin Y, Valassiadou K, Lewis S, Denley H. (2004) Investigation into the possible cause of subjective decreased sensory perception in the nipple-areola complex of women with macromastia. *Plast Reconstr Surg.* **113**(6):1598–1606. doi:10.1097/01.PRS.0000117190.00235.5C

39. Schreiber JE, Girotto JA, Mofid MM, Singh N, Nahabedian MY. (2004) Comparison study of nipple-areolar sensation after reduction mammaplasty. *Aesthet Surg J.* **24**(4):320–323. doi:10.1016/j.asj.2004.04.004

40. Schlenz I, Rigel S, Schemper M, Kuzbari R. (2005) Alteration of nipple and areola sensitivity by reduction mammaplasty: a prospective comparison of five techniques. *Plast Reconstr Surg.* **115**(3):743–751. doi:10.1097/01.PRS.0000152435.03538.43

41. Hall-Findlay E, Shestak K. (2015) Breast reduction. *Plast Reconstr Surg.* **136**(4):531e–544e. doi:10.1097/PRS.0000000000001622

42. Tairych GV, Kuzbari R, Rigel S, Todoroff BP, Schneider B, Deutinger M. (1998) Normal cutaneous sensibility of the breast. *Plast Reconstr Surg.* **102**(3):701–704. doi:10.1097/00006534-199809030-00013

43. Cruz-Korchin N, Korchin L. (2004) Breast-feeding after vertical mammaplasty with medial pedicle. *Plast Reconstr Surg.* **114**(4):890–894. doi:10.1097/01.PRS.0000133174.64330.CC

44. Strömbeck JO. (1971) Reduction mammaplasty. *Surg Clin North Am.* **51**(2):453–469. doi:10.1016/S0039-6109(16)39389-6

45. Davis GM, Ringler SL, Short K, Sherrick D, Bengtson BP. (1995) Reduction mammaplasty: long-term efficacy, morbidity, and patient satisfaction. *Plast Reconstr Surg.* **96**(5):1106–1110. doi:10.1097/00006534-199510000-00015

46. Schnur P, Schnur D, Petty P, Hanson T, Weaver M. (1997) Reduction mammaplasty: an outcome study. *Plast Reconstr Surg.* **100**:875–883. doi:10.1097/00006534-199709001-00008

47. Cruz-Korchin N, Korchin L. (2003) Vertical versus wise pattern breast reduction: patient satisfaction, revision rates, and complications. *Plast Reconstr Surg.* **112**:1573–1578. doi:10.1097/01.PRS.0000086736.61832.33

48. Fish JS, Bain JR, Levine R. (1994) Breast sensation following reduction mammaplasty. *Can J Plast Surg.* **2**(1):28–31. doi:10.1177/229255039400200102

49. Cunningham B, Gear A, Kerrigan C, Collins E. (2005) Analysis of breast reduction complications derived from the BRAVO study. *Plast Reconstr Surg.* **115**(6):1597–1604. doi:10.1097/01.PRS.0000160695.33457.DB

50. Hoffman S. (1986) Recurrent deformities following reduction mammaplasty and correction of breast asymmetry. *Plast Reconstr Surg.* **78**(1):55–62. doi:10.1097/00006534-198607000-00007

51. Spector J, Kleinerman R, Culliford AI, Karp N. (2006) The vertical reduction mammaplasty: a prospective analysis of patient outcomes. *Plast Reconstr Surg.* **117**(2):374–381. doi:10.1097/01.prs.0000197336.68801.8d

52. Thoma A, Ignacy TA, Duku EK, *et al.* (2013) Randomized controlled trial comparing health-related quality of life in patients undergoing vertical scar versus inverted T–shaped reduction mammaplasty. *Plast Reconstr Surg.* **132**(1):48e–60e. doi:10.1097/PRS.0b013e3182910cb0

53. American Society of Plastic Surgeons. (2018) Plastic surgery procedural statistics. https://www.plasticsurgery.org/documents/News/Statistics/2018/plastic-surgery-statistics-report-2018.pdf.

54. Blondeel PN, Hamdi M, Van de Sijpe KA, Van Landuyt KHI, Thiessen FEF, Monstrey SJM. (2003) The latero-central glandular pedicle technique for breast reduction. *Br J Plast Surg.* **56**(4):348–359. doi:10.1016/S0007-1226(03)00191-7

55. U.S. Food and Drug Administration. Medical device reports of breast implant-associated anaplastic large cell lymphoma. https://www.fda.gov/medical-devices/implants-and-prosthetics/breast-implants. Accessed February 12, 2017.

56. Gurunluoglu R, Kubek E, Arton J. (2013) Dual pedicle mastopexy technique for reorientation of volume and shape after subglandular and submuscular breast implant removal. *Eplasty.* **13**:e48. https://www.ncbi.nlm.nih.gov/pmc/articles/PMC3776568/. Accessed December 3, 2019.

57. Gurunluoglu R, Sacak B, Arton J. (2013) Outcomes analysis of patients undergoing autoaugmentation after breast implant removal. *Plast Reconstr Surg.* **132**(2):304–315. doi:10.1097/PRS.0b013e31829e7d9e

58. Hönig JF, Frey HP, Hasse FM, Hasselberg J. (2010) Inferior pedicle autoaugmentation mastopexy after breast implant removal. *Aesth Plast Surg.* **34**(4):447–454. doi:10.1007/s00266-010-9471-4

59. Graf RM, Closs Ono MC, Pace D, Balbinot P, Pazio ALB, de Paula DR. (2019) Breast autoaugmentation (mastopexy and lipofilling): an option for quitting breast implants. *Aesth Plast Surg.* **43**(5):1133–1141. doi:10.1007/s00266-019-01387-5

60. Mess SA. (2018) Lipoaugmentation following implant removal preferred by plastic surgeons and the general public. *Plast Reconstr Surg Glob Open.* **6**(8):e1882. doi:10.1097/GOX.0000000000001882

61. Rohrich RJ, Beran SJ, Restifo RJ, Copit SE. (1998) Aesthetic management of the breast following explantation: evaluation and mastopexy options. *Plast Reconstr Surg.* **101**(3):827–837. doi:10.1097/00006534-199803000-00039

62. Gonzales-Ulloa M. (1960) Correction of hypotrophy of the breast by means of exogenous material. *Plast Reconstr Surg Transplant Bull.* **25**:15–26. doi:10.1097/00006534-196001000-00002

63. Spear SL, Dayan J, Clements MW. (2009) Augmentation mastopexy. *Clin Plast Surg.* **36**(1):105–115. doi:10.1016/j.cps.2008.08.006

64. Spear S. (2003) Augmentation/mastopexy: "surgeon, beware." *Plast Reconstr Surg.* **112**(3):905–906. doi:10.1097/01.PRS.0000072257.66189.3E

65. Hoffman S. (2004) Some thoughts on augmentation/mastopexy and medical malpractice. *Plast Reconstr Surg.* **113**(6):1892–1893. doi:10.1097/01.PRS.0000119889.57805.D3

66. Stevens WG, Stoker DA, Freeman ME, Quardt SM, Hirsch EM, Cohen R. (2006) Is one-stage breast augmentation with mastopexy safe and effective? A review of 186 primary cases. *Aesthet Surg J.* **26**(6):674–681. doi:10.1016/j.asj.2006.10.003

67. Hickman DM. (2011) Application of the goes double-skin peri-areolar mastopexy with and without implants: a 14-year experience. *J Plast Reconstr Aesthetic Surg.* **64**(2):164–173. doi:10.1016/j.bjps.2009.11.033

68. Gonzalez R. (2012) The PAM method — periareolar augmentation mastopexy: a personal approach to treat hypoplastic breast with moderate ptosis. *Aesthet Surg J.* **32**(2):175–185. doi:10.1177/1090820X11431578

69. Calobrace MB, Herdt DR, Cothron KJ. (2013) Simultaneous augmentation/mastopexy: a retrospective 5-year review of 332 consecutive cases. *Plast Reconstr Surg.* **131**(1):145–156. doi:10.1097/PRS.0b013e318272bf86

70. Beale EW, Ramanadham S, Harrison B, Rasko Y, Armijo B, Rohrich RJ. (2014) Achieving predictability in augmentation mastopexy. *Plast Reconstr Surg.* **133**(3):284e. doi:10.1097/PRS.0000000000000079

71. Doshier LJ, Eagan SL, Shock LA, Henry SL, Colbert SH, Puckett CL. (2016) The subtleties of success in simultaneous augmentation-mastopexy. *Plast Reconstr Surg.* **138**:585–592. doi:10.1097/PRS.0000000000002517

72. White CP, Farhang Khoee H, Kattan AE, Farrokhyar F, Hynes NM. (2013) Breast reduction scars: a prospective survey of patient preferences. *Aesthet Surg J.* **33**(6):817–821. doi:10.1177/1090820X13495868

73. Marshall CD, Hu MS, Leavitt T, Barnes LA, Lorenz HP, Longaker MT. (2018) Cutaneous scarring: basic science, current treatments, and future directions. *Adv Wound Care.* **7**(2):29–45. doi:10.1089/wound.2016.0696

74. Hever P, Cavale N, Pasha T. (2019) A retrospective comparison of 3M™ micropore™ with other common dressings in cosmetic breast surgery. *J Plast Reconstr Aesthetic Surg.* **72**(3):424–426. doi:10.1016/j.bjps.2018.11.007

75. Mîra A, Carton A-K, Muller S, Payan Y. (2018) A biomechanical breast model evaluated with respect to MRI data collected in three different positions. *Clin Biomech.* **60**:191–199. doi:10.1016/j.clinbiomech.2018.10.020

76. Veiga DF, Damasceno CAV, Veiga-Filho J, *et al.* (2016) Dressing wear time after breast reconstruction: a randomized clinical trial. *PLoS One.* **11**(12):e0166356. doi:10.1371/journal.pone.0166356

77. Webster J, Liu Z, Norman G, *et al.* (2019) Negative pressure wound therapy for surgical wounds healing by primary closure. *Cochrane Database Syst Rev.* **3**:CD009261. doi:10.1002/14651858. CD009261.pub4

78. Courtiss EH, Goldwyn RM. (1976) Breast sensation before and after plastic surgery. *Plast Reconstr Surg.* **58**(1):1–13. doi:10.1097/00006534-197607000-00001

79. Ziolkowski N, Kitto SC, Jeong D, *et al.* (2019) Psychosocial and quality of life impact of scars in the surgical, traumatic and burn populations: a scoping review protocol. *BMJ Open.* **9**(6):e021289. doi:10.1136/bmjopen-2017-021289

80. Seago M, Shumaker PR, Spring LK, *et al.* (2019) Laser treatment of traumatic scars and contractures: 2020 international consensus recommendations. *Lasers Surg Med.* doi:10.1002/lsm.23201

81. Manstein D, Herron GS, Sink RK, Tanner H, Anderson RR. (2004) Fractional photothermolysis: a new concept for cutaneous remodeling using microscopic patterns of thermal injury. *Lasers Surg Med.* **34**(5):426–438. doi:10.1002/lsm.20048

82. Shin JU, Gantsetseg D, Jung JY, Jung I, Shin S, Lee JH. (2014) Comparison of non-ablative and ablative fractional laser treatments in a postoperative scar study. *Lasers Surg Med.* **46**(10):741–749. doi:10.1002/lsm.22297

83. Lin JY, Warger WC, Izikson L, Anderson RR, Tannous Z. (2011) A prospective, randomized controlled trial on the efficacy of fractional photothermolysis on scar remodeling. *Lasers Surg Med.* **43**(4):265–272. doi:10.1002/lsm.21061

84. Clementoni MT, Pedrelli V, Zaccaria G, Pontini P, Motta LR, Azzopardi EA. (2020) New developments for fractional Co2 resurfacing for skin rejuvenation and scar reduction. *Facial Plast Surg Clin.* **28**(1):17–28. doi:10.1016/j.fsc.2019.09.002

85. Issler-Fisher AC, Waibel JS, Donelan MB. (2017) Laser modulation of hypertrophic scars: technique and practice. *Clin Plast Surg.* **44**(4):757–766. doi:10.1016/j.cps.2017.05.007

86. Hædersdal M, Sakamoto FH, Farinelli WA, Doukas AG, Tam J, Anderson RR. (2010) Fractional CO2 laser-assisted drug delivery. *Lasers Surg Med.* **42**(2):113–122. doi:10.1002/lsm.20860

87. Sklar LR, Burnett CT, Waibel JS, Moy RL, Ozog DM. (2014) Laser assisted drug delivery: a review of an evolving technology. *Lasers Surg Med.* **46**(4):249–262. doi:10.1002/lsm.22227

88. Waibel JS, Wulkan AJ, Shumaker PR. (2013) Treatment of hypertrophic scars using laser and laser assisted corticosteroid delivery. *Lasers Surg Med.* **45**(3):135–140. doi:10.1002/lsm.22120

89. Keaney TC, Tanzi E, Alster T. (2016) Comparison of 532 nm potassium titanyl phosphate laser and 595 nm pulsed dye laser in the treatment of erythematous surgical scars: a randomized, controlled, open-label study. *Dermatol Surg.* **42**(1):70. doi:10.1097/DSS.0000000000000582

90. Kuo Y-R, Wu W-S, Wang F-S. (2007) Flashlamp pulsed-dye laser suppressed TGF-β1 expression and proliferation in cultured keloid fibroblasts is mediated by MAPK pathway. *Lasers Surg Med.* **39**(4):358–364. doi:10.1002/lsm.20489

91. Manuskiatti W, Fitzpatrick RE. (2002) Treatment response of keloidal and hypertrophic sternotomy scars: comparison among intralesional corticosteroid, 5-fluorouracil, and 585-nm flashlamp-pumped pulsed-dye laser treatments. *Arch Dermatol.* **138**(9):1149–1155. doi:10.1001/archderm. 138.9.1149

92. Ouyang H, Li G, Lei Y, Gold MH, Tan J. (2018) Comparison of the effectiveness of pulsed dye laser vs pulsed dye laser combined with ultrapulse fractional CO2 laser in the treatment of immature red hypertrophic scars. *J Cosmet Dermatol.* **17**(1):54–60. doi:10.1111/jocd.12487

93. Asilian A, Darougheh A, Shariati F. (2006) New combination of triamcinolone, 5-fluorouracil, and pulsed-dye laser for treatment of keloid and hypertrophic scars. *Dermatol Surg.* **32**(7):907–915. doi:10.1111/j.1524-4725.2006.32195.x

94. Artzi O, Koren A, Niv R, Mehrabi JN, Friedman O. (2019) The scar bane, without the pain: a new approach in the treatment of elevated scars: thermomechanical delivery of topical triamcinolone acetonide and 5-fluorouracil. *Dermatol Ther (Heidelb).* **9**(2):321–326. doi:10.1007/s13555-019-0298-x

95. Artzi O, Koren A, Niv R, Mehrabi JN, Mashiah J, Friedman O. (2020) A new approach in the treatment of pediatric hypertrophic burn scars: tixel-associated topical triamcinolone acetonide and 5-fluorouracil delivery. *J Cosmet Dermatol.* **19**:131–134. doi:10.1111/jocd.13192

96. Magnani LR, Schweiger ES. (2014) Fractional CO2 lasers for the treatment of atrophic acne scars: a review of the literature. *J Cosmet Laser Ther.* **16**(2):48–56. doi:10.3109/14764172.2013.854639

97. Rkein A, Ozog D, Waibel JS. (2014) Treatment of atrophic scars with fractionated CO2 laser facilitating delivery of topically applied poly-L-lactic acid. *Dermatol Surg.* **40**(6):624. doi:10.1111/dsu.0000000000000010

98. Bach D, Garcia M, Eisen D. (2012) Hyperpigmented burn scar improved with a fractionated 1550 nm non-ablative laser. *Dermatol Online J.* **18**(7):12.

99. Koren A, Niv R, Cohen S, Artzi O. (2019) A 1064-nm Neodymium-doped yttrium aluminum garnet picosecond laser for the treatment of hyperpigmented scars. *Dermatol Surg.* **45**(5):725. doi:10.1097/DSS.0000000000001917

100. Siadat AH, Rezaei R, Asilian A, *et al.* (2015) Repigmentation of hypopigmented scars using combination of fractionated carbon dioxide laser with topical latanoprost vs. fractionated carbon dioxide laser alone. *Indian J Dermatol.* **60**(4):364–368. doi:10.4103/0019-5154.160481

101. Massaki ABMN, Fabi SG, Fitzpatrick R. (2012) Repigmentation of hypopigmented scars using an erbium-doped 1,550-nm fractionated laser and topical bimatoprost. *Dermatol Surg.* **38**(7 pt 1):995–1001. doi:10.1111/j.1524-4725.2012.02389.x

102. Schmidt M, Serror K, Chaouat M, Mimoun M, Boccara D. (2018) Prise en charge des cicatrices hypopigmentées post-brûlure. *Ann Chir Plast Esth.* **63**(3):246–254. doi:10.1016/j.anplas.2017.10.006

103. Karmisholt KE, Haerskjold A, Karlsmark T, Waibel J, Paasch U, Haedersdal M. (2018) Early laser intervention to reduce scar formation — a systematic review. *J Eur Acad Dermatol Venereol.* **32**(7):1099–1110. doi:10.1111/jdv.14856

104. Park KY, Oh IY, Seo SJ, Kang KH, Park SJ. (2013) Appropriate timing for thyroidectomy scar treatment using a 1,550-nm fractional erbium-glass laser. *Dermatol Surg.* **39**(12):1827–1834. doi:10.1111/dsu.12355

105. Zhang Y, Liu Y, Cai B, *et al.* (2019) Improvement of surgical scars by early intervention with carbon dioxide fractional laser. *Lasers Surg Med.* doi:10.1002/lsm.23129

106. Karmisholt KE, Wenande E, Thaysen-Petersen D, Philipsen PA, Paasch U, Haedersdal M. (2018) Early intervention with non-ablative fractional laser to improve cutaneous scarring — a randomized controlled trial on the impact of intervention time and fluence levels. *Lasers Surg Med.* **50**(1):28–36. doi:10.1002/lsm.22707

107. Safra T, Shehadeh W, Koren A, *et al.* (2019) Early intervention with pulse dye and CO2 ablative fractional lasers to improve cutaneous scarring post-lumpectomy: a randomized controlled trial on the impact of intervention on final cosmesis. *Lasers Med Sci.* **34**(9):1881–1887. doi:10.1007/s10103-019-02788-3

LIST OF ABBREVIATIONS

AFR	Ablative Fractional Resurfacing
ASPS	American Society of Plastic Surgeons
BEP	Borenstein Explantation–Pexy
BMI	Body Mass Index
FACL	Fractional Ablative CO_2 Laser
IMF	Inframammary Fold
IPL	Intense Pulse Laser
KTP	Potassium Titanyl Phosphate
LADD	Laser-Assisted Drug Delivery
NAC	Nipple–Areola Complex
NAFL	Non-Ablative Fractional Laser
NAFR	Non-Ablative Fractional Resurfacing
PDL	Pulsed Dye Laser
PLLA	Poly-l-Lactic Acid
SL	Shock LA
SSI	Surgical Site Infection

Index

ablative fractional resurfacing, 69
adolescents, 17
advanced scar treatments, 67
arteries, 1
Artzi, 67
augmentation and mastopexy, 49
augmentation and multi-level mastopexy, 49
augmentations, 44

BIA-ALCL, 44
blood supply, 3
Borenstein maneuver, 28, 44, 50
breast, 1
breast shape, 63
but they usually have reasonable expectations, 17

can be performed safely and effectively, 49
circummammary ligament, 1
CO_2 laser, 68
complications, 63
Cooper ligaments, 1
correction of ptosis, 18

deflated breast, 24
dermal flaps, 28
dissection, 2

expectations, 17
explantation–pexy, 41

foundations, 9
fractional lasers, 68
fundamentals, 9

Go On, I Am Listening, 17

healing, 64
hypertrophic, 67

implant extrusion, 55
inferior and lateral vector, 9
irrigation and careful hemostasis, 44

KTP, 72

laser-assisted drug delivery (LADD), 68
lateral capsule to the IMF, 44
long-term, 63

mastopexy, 41
minimal tension sutures, 9
minimize scarring, 67
motivations, 17
multi-level, 9

nerves, 1
nipple sensitivity, 17

older women, 18
opposing vectors, 49
Out With the Old, 41

partially de-epithelialized, 11
pectoralis, 1
pillar sutures, 28
Postoperational Breast Support, 59
postoperative pain, 17

post-surgical scars, 67
pre-surgical markings are only rough guides, 9
prostaglandin, 72
pulsed dye laser (PDL), 68

reduce the risk, 55

scar pattern, 59
scarring, 59
secure the foundation, 23
significant lateral vector, 23
skin quality, 59
Stand By Me, 63
sterile porous tape, 59
stress, 67
superficial fascia, 1
supported throughout its height, 9
surgical anatomy, 1

taking the stress out of the breast, 49
tension-free skin closure, 12
The Paper Bra, 59
two thin dermal flaps, 50

unavoidable scars, 18
unrealistic expectations, 18

vertical scar reduction, 23

widening of the scar, 65
With Your Own, 41
wound dehiscence, 55

younger patients, 17

CPSIA information can be obtained
at www.ICGtesting.com
Printed in the USA
BVHW010908230720
584324BV00001B/2